# USMLE

# RECALL SERIES EDITOR

**LORNE H. BLACKBOURNE, MD**
Trauma, Burn, and Critical Care Surgeon
San Antonio, Texas

# USMLE STEP 2 RECALL

Editor

## Michael W. Ryan, MD, MS
Gastroenterology Fellow
Saint Louis University School of Medicine
Division of Gastroenterology and Hepatology
St. Louis, Missouri

Lippincott Williams & Wilkins
a Wolters Kluwer business
Philadelphia · Baltimore · New York · London
Buenos Aires · Hong Kong · Sydney · Tokyo

*Acquisitions Editor:* Donna Balado
*Managing Editor:* Cheryl W. Stringfellow
*Marketing Manager:* Jennifer Kuklinski
*Production Editor:* Jennifer D.W. Glazer
*Designer:* Doug Smock
*Compositor:* International Typesetting and Composition
*Printer:* R.R. Donnelley & Sons—Crawfordsville

Copyright © 2007 Lippincott Williams & Wilkins

351 West Camden Street
Baltimore, MD 21201

530 Walnut Street
Philadelphia, PA 19106

*Printed in the United States of America*

**Library of Congress Cataloging-in-Publication Data**

Ryan, Michael W.
  USMLE step 2 recall / Michael W. Ryan.
    p. ; cm.—(Recall series)
  Includes index.
    ISBN-13: 978-0-7817-8850-2
    ISBN-10: 0-7817-8850-1
    1. Clinical medicine—Case studies.   2. Physicians—Licenses—United States—
Examinations—Study guides.  I. Title.  II. Title: USMLE step two recall.
III. Series.
    [DNLM:  1. Medicine—Case Reports.   2. Medicine—Examination Questions.
3. Diagnosis, Differential—Case Reports.   4. Diagnosis, Differential—Examination
Questions.    W 18.2 R989u 2007]
RC66.R93 2007
616'.0076—dc22

                                                 2006026413

To purchase additional copies of this book, call our customer service department at
**(800) 638-3030** or fax orders to **(301) 223-2320.** International customers should call
**(301) 223-2300.**

***Visit Lippincott Williams & Wilkins on the Internet: http://www.LWW.com.*** Lippincott
Williams & Wilkins customer service representatives are available from 8:30 am to
6:00 pm, EST.

                                  06  07  08  09  10
                1  2  3  4  5  6  7  8  9  10

# Dedication

*This book is dedicated to my loving wife, Krista, and my sons, Brady and Parker.*

# Preface

Purchase this book if you are looking for a case-based book that reinforces important content stressed within the USMLE Step 2 exam through a question and answer format.

The case-based approach was chosen to simulate real questions on the exam. The active-learning question-and-answer format following the patient presentation was chosen to ensure rapid comprehension of essential material needed to do well on the Step 2 exam. Your confidence and mastery of the material will increase dramatically with each interactive case-based review session.

The content was chosen after comparing the official USMLE Step 2 study outline to the key points stressed in review questions and by students with high scores on the exam. Only the essential information is covered here.

Congratulations on purchasing an essential active-learning review tool for the USMLE Step 2 exam!

# The Test

The USMLE Step 2 exam is now composed of the clinical knowledge (CK) and the clinical skills (CS) parts. The CS part is a 1-day live exam on 12 standardized patients. The CK exam is a 1-day multiple-choice computer-based examination. The information learned from this book will be useful for each part of the exam. It teaches pattern recognition for diseases tested in multiple-choice and live patient presentations. For further information regarding the CS exam, please visit *www.usmle.org*.

The CK exam is a computer-based test taken at Prometric Test Centers using FROG software. It is a 9-hour exam with 368 multiple-choice questions broken up into eight 60-minute blocks with 45 minutes of break time in between. An additional 15 minutes can be used during the 9-hour block to go through the FROG software tutorial. By visiting *www.usmle.org* you can become familiar with the FROG software prior to the test date. This will allow you to bypass the tutorial and an additional 15 minutes will be added to your break time. Once a question block is started, it must be completed within the time provided. Breaks may only be taken between question blocks. If you complete a question block early, this will be added to your break time.

Multiple-choice single-best-answer formats comprise over 80% of the exam questions. Single-best-answer matching sets comprise the remaining exam questions. This format typically has two questions related to a common topic with 4 to 26 possible answers to chose from. You may practice the exam question formats by visiting *www.usmle.org*.

To register for the exam, visit *www.nbme.org* and print out an application or apply on-line. You will need to specify a 3-month block of time during which you plan to take the examination. Once your application has been approved, you will be mailed an orange permit with your ID number on it. Do not lose this permit. The ID number is required to schedule an exam date with a Prometric Test Center and the orange permit must be provided on the day of the exam along with a photo ID to take the exam. For additional information and to schedule your exam date, please visit *www.prometric.com*.

Rest assured that the case-based, rapid-fire question-and-answer format in USMLE Step 2 Recall will provide you with the necessary fund of knowledge needed to excel on this examination.

# Contents

# Common Abbreviations

| | |
|---|---|
| ā | Before |
| AAA | Abdominal aortic aneurysm, "triple A" |
| ABD | Army battle dressing |
| ABG | Arterial blood gas |
| ABI | Ankle to brachial index |
| ACE | Angiotensin converting enzyme |
| Ach | Acetylcholine |
| ACTH | Adrenocorticotropic hormone |
| AF | Atrial fibrillation |
| AKA | Above-the-knee amputation |
| a.k.a. | Also known as |
| AMI | Acute myocardial infarction |
| AML | Acute myclogenous leukemia |
| ALL | Acute lymphoblastic leukemia |
| ALT | Alanine aminotransference |
| Ao | Aorta |
| APR | Abdominoperineal resection |
| AR | Aortic regurgitation |
| ARDS | Acute respiratory distress syndrome |
| AS | Aortic stenosis |
| ASA | Aspirin |
| AST | Aspartate transaminase |
| AVM | Arteriovenous malformation |
| AXR | Abdominal x-ray |
| B1 | Billroth 1 gastroduodenostomy |
| B2 | Billroth 2 gastrojejunostomy |
| BCC | Basal cell carcinoma |
| BCP | Birth control pill |

| | |
|---|---|
| **BE** | Barium enema |
| **BIH** | Bilateral inguinal hernia |
| **BKA** | Below-the-knee amputation |
| **BPH** | Benign prostatic hypertrophy |
| **BRBPR** | Bright red blood per rectum |
| **BS** | Bowel sounds, breath sounds, blood sugar |
| **BSE** | Breast self-examination |
| **c̄** | With |
| **CA** | Cancer |
| **CABG** | Coronary artery bypass graft ("CABBAGE") |
| **CAD** | Coronary artery disease |
| **CAP** | Community-acquired pneumonia |
| **CBC** | Complete blood cell count |
| **CBD** | Common bile duct |
| **CHF** | Congestive heart failure |
| **CML** | Chronic myelogenous leukemia |
| **C/O** | Complains of |
| **COPD** | Chronic obstructive pulmonary disease |
| **CP** | Chest pain |
| **CRC** | Colorectal cancer |
| **CTA** | Clear to auscultation |
| **CVA** | Cerebral vascular accident, costovertebral angle |
| **CVP** | Central venous pressure |
| **CXR** | Chest x-ray |
| **Dx** | Diagnosis |
| **DDx** | Differential diagnosis |
| **DI** | Diabetes insipidus |
| **DJD** | Degenerative joint disease |

| | |
|---|---|
| **DM** | Diabetes mellitus, dermatomyositis |
| **DOE** | Dyspnea on exertion |
| **DP** | Dorsalis pedalis |
| **DPL** | Diagnostic peritoneal lavage |
| **DPC** | Delayed primary closure |
| **DT** | Delirium tremens |
| **DVT** | Deep venous thrombosis |
| **EBL** | Estimated blood loss |
| **EKG** | Electrocardiogram |
| **ECMO** | Extracorporeal membrane oxygenation |
| **EGD** | Esophagogastroduodenoscopy (UGI scope) |
| **EOMI** | Extraocular muscles intact |
| **ERCP** | Endoscopic retrograde cholangiopancreatography |
| **ETOH** | Alcohol |
| **EUA** | Exam under anesthesia |
| **FAP** | Familial adenomatous polyposis |
| **FAST** | Focused abdominal sonogram for trauma |
| **FEN** | Fluids, electrolytes, nutrition |
| **FNA** | Fine needle aspiration |
| **FOBT** | Fecal occult blood test |
| **GBS** | Guillain-Barré syndrome |
| **GCS** | Glasgow Coma Scale |
| **GERD** | Gastroesophageal reflux disease |
| **GET(A)** | General endotracheal (anesthesia) |
| **GU** | Genitourinary |
| **HCM** | Hypertrophic cardiomyopathy |
| **HCT** | Hematocrit |
| **HEENT** | Head, eyes, ears, nose, and throat |

| | |
|---|---|
| **HG** | Hemorrhagic gastritis |
| **HO** | House officer |
| **HTN** | Hypertension |
| **IABP** | Intra-aortic balloon pump |
| **IBD** | Inflammatory bowel disease |
| **ICU** | Intensive care unit |
| **I & D** | Incision and drainage |
| **IDU** | Injection drug user |
| **IE** | Infective endocarditis |
| **ILD** | Interstitial lung disease |
| **I & O** | Ins and outs, in and out |
| **IMV** | Intermittent mandatory ventilation |
| **IPF** | Idiopathic pulmonary fibrosis |
| **IVC** | Inferior vena cava |
| **IVF** | Intravenous fluids |
| **IVP** | Intravenous pyelography |
| **IVPB** | Intravenous piggyback |
| **JVD** | Jugular venous distention |
| **(L)** | Left |
| **LAP APPY** | Laparoscopic appendectomy |
| **LAP CHOLE** | Laparoscopic cholecystectomy |
| **LDH** | Lactate dehydrogenase |
| **LE** | Lower extremity |
| **LES** | Lower esophageal sphincter |
| **LIH** | Left inguinal hernia |
| **LLQ** | Left lower quadrant |
| **LR** | Lactated Ringer's |
| **LUQ** | Left upper quadrant |
| **LVH** | Left ventricular hypertrophy |
| **MAE** | Moving all extremities |

| | |
|---|---|
| **MAST** | Military antishock trousers |
| **MEN** | Multiple endocrine neoplasia |
| **MI** | Myocardial infarction |
| **MIBG** | $^{131}$I-metaiodobenzylguanidine |
| **MSO$_4$** | Morphine sulfate |
| **NGT** | Nasogastric tube |
| **NPO** | Nothing per os |
| **NS** | Normal saline |
| **OBR** | Ortho bowel routine |
| **OCTOR** | On call to OR |
| **OOB** | Out of bed |
| **ORIF** | Open reduction internal fixation |
| **p̄** | After |
| **PCa** | Prostate cancer |
| **PCWP** | Pulmonary capillary wedge pressure |
| **PE** | Pulmonary embolism, Physical examination |
| **PEEP** | Positive end-expiratory pressure |
| **PEG** | Percutaneous endoscopic gastrostomy (via EGD and skin incision) |
| **PERRL** | Pupils equal and react to light |
| **PFT** | Pulmonary function tests |
| **PICC** | Peripherally inserted central catheter |
| **PGV** | Proximal gastric vagotomy (i.e., leaves fibers to pylorus intact to preserve emptying) |
| **PID** | Pelvic inflammatory disease |
| **PMI** | Posterior myocardial infarction |
| **PO** | Per os (by mouth) |
| **POD** | Postoperative day |
| **PPD** | Purified protein derivative |

| | |
|---|---|
| **PT** | Physical therapy, Patient, Posterior tibial |
| **PTH** | Parathyroid hormone |
| **PR** | Per rectum |
| **PRN** | As needed: literally "pro re nata" |
| **PTC** | Percutaneous transhepatic cholangiogram (dye injected via a catheter through skin and into dilated intrahepatic bile duct) |
| **PTCA** | Percutaneous transluminal coronary angioplasty |
| **PTSD** | Posttraumatic stress disorder |
| **PTU** | Propylthiouracil |
| **PTX** | pneumothorax |
| **PUD** | Peptic ulcer disease |
| **PVE** | Prosthetic valve endocarditis |
| **q̄** | Every |
| **QD** | Every day |
| **QOD** | Every other day |
| **Ⓡ** | Right |
| **RIH** | Right inguinal hernia |
| **RLQ** | Right lower quadrant |
| **RTC** | Return to clinic |
| **RUQ** | Right upper quadrant |
| **Rx** | Treatment |
| **s̄** | Without |
| **SBO** | Small bowel obstruction |
| **SCC** | Squamous cell carcinoma |
| **SCD** | Sequential compression device |
| **SIADH** | Syndrome of inappropriate antidiuretic hormone |
| **SICU** | Surgical intensive care unit |
| **SLE** | Systemic lupus erythematosus |

| | |
|---|---|
| **SOAP** | Subjective, objective, assessment, and plan |
| **STSG** | Split thickness skin graft |
| **SVC** | Superior vena cava |
| **Sx** | Symptoms |
| **T & C** | Type and cross |
| **T & S** | Type and screen |
| **TB** | Tuberculosis |
| **TCA** | Tricyclic antidepressant |
| **TEE** | Transesophageal echocardiography |
| **Tmax** | Maximal temperature |
| **TPN** | Total parenteral nutrition |
| **TSH** | Thyroid-stimulating hormone |
| **TURP** | Transurethral resection of the prostate |
| **UE** | Upper extremity |
| **UGI** | Upper gastrointestinal |
| **UO** | Urine output |
| **URTI** | Upper respiratory tract infection |
| **US** | Ultrasound |
| **UTI** | Urinary tract infection |
| **VAD** | Ventricular assist device |
| **VOCTOR** | Void on call to OR |
| **VSD** | Ventricular septal defect |
| $\mathbf{W \rightarrow D}$ | Wet-to-dry dressing |
| **XRT** | X-ray therapy |
| **ZE** | Zollinger-Ellison syndrome |
| $-$ | No, negative |
| $+$ | Yes, positive |
| $\uparrow$ | Increase, more |
| $\downarrow$ | Decrease, less |
| $<$ | Less than |
| $>$ | Greater than |

# 1     Cardiology

## HYPERTENSION

### CASE I

*An 11-year-old boy presents to you after being found to have elevated blood pressure at a community health fair. You confirm elevated blood pressure in his arm and are impressed with asymmetric pulses in the arms, weak leg pulses, and a harsh systolic murmur between the scapulae.*

| | |
|---|---|
| **What should you do next on your physical exam?** | Take the blood pressure in the legs |
| **Why? What do you suspect?** | Coarctation of the aorta |
| **What childhood disease is associated with this?** | Turner's syndrome |
| **Blood pressure in legs is normal. What's your probable diagnosis?** | Coarctation of the aorta |
| **What causes it?** | A localized narrowing of the aortic arch just distal to the origin of the left subclavian artery |
| **How does it present?** | Usually with asymptomatic hypertension |
| **What signs are found on physical exam?** | Asymmetric pulses in the upper extremities with absent or weak pulses in the lower extremities; harsh systolic murmur between the scapulae |
| **What additional tests should you order to support your diagnosis?** | EKG, CXR |

| | |
|---|---|
| **What findings do you expect on:** | |
| **EKG?** | Left ventricular hypertrophy |
| **CXR?** | Rib notching on CXR |
| **What test will confirm the diagnosis?** | Arteriogram or Doppler echo |
| **What is the treatment?** | Surgery |

## CASE 2

*A 44-year-old female with history of gout, chronic hepatitis C, and diverticulosis presents with weakness, fatigue, easy bruising, puffy cheeks, and new onset acne and hypertension.*

| | |
|---|---|
| **What's most likely causing her hypertension?** | Cushing's syndrome |
| **What causes it?** | Adrenal overproduction (adrenal tumors or from ectopic ACTH stimulation from an oat-cell lung cancer) and exogenously administered steroid (most common) |
| **When does Cushing's syndrome become Cushing's disease?** | When the excess cortisol is caused by abnormally increased secretion of adrenocorticotropic hormone (ACTH) secreted by the pituitary (pituitary adenoma) |
| **What are the symptoms?** | Weakness, fatigue, moodiness, and easy bruising |
| **What are the signs?** | Hypertension and cushingoid appearance (truncal obesity, abdominal striae, impaired glucose tolerance, hirsutism, acne, and osteoporosis) |
| **What lab values suggest the diagnosis?** | Increased serum, urinary cortisol, and cortisol metabolites; hypokalemia and mild hyperglycemia (effects of cortisol) |

| | |
|---|---|
| **What diagnostic test should you order?** | 1 mg overnight dexamethasone suppression test and 24-hour urinary-free cortisol |
| **What is the treatment for pituitary tumors?** | Transphenoid microadenectomy |
| **What is the treatment for adrenal tumors and oat-cell lung cancer?** | Surgical resection, if possible |

## CASE 3

*A 49-year-old overweight diabetic male presents to your clinic after an extensive evaluation in another state for new onset of hypertension (HTN). His prior physician ruled out secondary causes of HTN including hyperaldosteronism, pheochromocytoma, renal parenchymal hypertension, renovascular disease, coarctation of the aorta, and Cushing syndrome. Currently, his BP is 144/83, pulse 76, and creatinine 1.0 on hydrochlorothiazide.*

| | |
|---|---|
| **What type of hypertension does he have?** | Essential hypertension |
| **How was the diagnosis made?** | BP $\geq$ 125/75 mm Hg on two occasions after secondary causes ruled out |
| **What is essential hypertension?** | The most common (~95% of cases) form of hypertension after secondary causes ruled out |
| **What are his risk factors?** | Age, diabetes, and overweight |
| **Name other known risk factors** | Kidney disease, physical inactivity, consumption of excessive amounts of alcohol |
| **What physical findings on exam would support chronic uncontrolled hypertension?** | Hypertensive retinopathy, laterally displaced PMI, and/or $S_4$ gallop |
| **Is his BP currently under control?** | No |
| **What's his goal BP?** | <125/75 |

| | |
|---|---|
| **What's your treatment strategy?** | Lifestyle modifications and antihypertensives |
| **Describe the lifestyle modifications** | Aerobic exercise, weight loss if overweight, dietary sodium restriction, alcohol <2 drinks per day |
| **What is a commonly used first-line antihypertensive?** | Hydrochlorothiazide (patient already on) |
| **What antihypertensive class should be considered in the following patients?** | |
| **Diabetics (this patient) and patients with controlled heart failure** | Angiotensin-converting enzyme (ACE) inhibitors |
| **Underlying coronary artery disease (CAD) or history of myocardial infarction (MI)** | β-blockers |
| **What other antihypertensives are available?** | Angiotensin receptor antagonists, α-blockers, calcium antagonists, sympatholytic and direct vasodilator drugs |
| **How many drugs are often needed to control blood pressure?** | 3 or more, to attain goal BP levels |
| **Why is it important to control BP?** | To decrease risk of kidney insufficiency or failure, left ventricular hypertrophy, heart failure, myocardial infarction, and/or peripheral arterial disease |

## CASE 4

*A 35-year-old male with uncontrolled hypertension on 4 medications presents to your office for follow-up after addition of the fourth medication. His blood pressure remains elevated at 155/90. His serum chemistry panel has routinely shown mildly low potassium which has not corrected with potassium supplementation.*

| | |
|---|---|
| **What should you suspect?** | Hyperaldosteronism |
| **What were the clues?** | Uncontrolled hypertension on multiple agents with hypokalemia |
| **Who is at risk?** | Typically persons between the ages of 30 and 50 years, with women affected more often than men |
| **What causes primary hyperaldosteronism?** | Autonomous secretion of aldosterone from the adrenal gland as a consequence of either a solitary adenoma (most common) or less commonly hyperplasia of both adrenal glands |
| **What screeing test should you order to workup hyperaldosteronism?** | Morning plasma aldosterone:renin ratio |
| **What is a positive screening test?** | Ratio >25 with an elevated plasma aldosterone level |
| **How is the diagnosis confirmed?** | Inability of intravenous or oral salt-loading to suppress 24-hour urinary excretion of aldosterone to <14 μg, or inability of plasma aldosterone ratio to suppress to <30 after 50 mg oral captopril |
| **What imaging tests should be ordered?** | CT or MRI scanning is preferred for localization and determining type of adrenal pathology, although adrenal vein sampling and adrenal NP-59 scans can help localize site of autonomous production. |
| **How is primary hyperaldosteronism treated?** | Medical or surgical (unilateral adrenalectomy) therapies |
| **What are the indications for surgical therapy?** | Unilateral adenoma in a good surgical candidate |

| What are the indications for medical therapy? | Unilateral adenoma in a poor surgical candidate and bilateral adrenal hyperplasia |
| --- | --- |
| What medical therapies are useful? | Thiazide and potassium-sparing diuretics—spironolactone, potassium supplements, and calcium antagonists are especially useful along with other antihypertensive agents and dietary sodium restriction. |

## CASE 5

*A 38-year-old male presents to your clinic with history of labile hypertension unresponsive to 4 commonly prescribed antihypertensives. He is adamant that he has been taking all his medications as prescribed and has new complaints of episodic sweating, headache, and rapid heart rate. At first, he thought he might have the flu, but now he's not sure.*

| What do you suspect? | Pheochromocytoma |
| --- | --- |
| Why? | Episodic headache, sweating, and tachycardia is the classic triad of symptoms for pheochromocytoma. |
| What relatively common conditions might pheochromocytoma be confused with? | Labile hypertension with hyperdynamic circulation, thyrotoxicosis, ingestion of sympathomimetic drugs, and abrupt discontinuation of sympatholytic drugs causing rebound hypertension |
| What other diseases is pheochromocytoma associated with? | Von Hippel-Lindau's and neurofibromatosis, multiple endocrine neoplasia (MEN) type 2A and 2B |
| What causes it? | A paraganglioma tumor arising from chromaffin cells in the adrenal medulla that secretes catecholamines—norepinephrine, epinephrine, dopamine—either continuously or episodically |

| | |
|---|---|
| **What screening tests should you order?** | Plasma metanephrines:creatinine ratio, plasma catecholamines, timed urine collections for metanephrines, metanephrines:creatinine urine catecholamines, and 3-methoxy-4-hydroxymandelic acid (VMA) |
| **Are there differences among the screening tests?** | 24-hour urinary metanephrine:creatinine ratio is more specific than urinary metanephrines (fewer false positives) and plasma metanephrine:creatinine ratio is more sensitive than plasma catecholamines. |
| **What's the next step after a positive screening test?** | Image by MRI or CT to locate the pheochromocytoma |
| **Which imaging modality is more sensitive for extra-adrenal pheochromocytomas?** | MRI |
| **What other tests are useful in localizing pheochromocytoma?** | $^{123}$I- or $^{131}$I-metaiodobenzylguanidine (MIBG) scintigraphy |
| **What's the treatment?** | Pre-operative α-adrenergic blockade phenoxybenzamine (dibenzyline) followed by surgical resection |

## CASE 6

*A 55-year-old diabetic female with history of 30 pack years smoking and refractory hypertension follows up in your clinic after addition of an ACE inhibitor to her antihypertensive regimen. You review the chemistry panel taken 2 weeks after starting the ACE inhibitor and are surprised to find the serum creatinine has risen from 0.8 to 1.5.*

| | |
|---|---|
| **What other diagnosis should be considered?** | Renal parenchymal hypertension |
| **What is it?** | The most common form of secondary or surgically curable hypertension occurring as a consequence of critical stenosis of one or both renal arteries |

| | |
|---|---|
| **What are the most common causes of renovascular hypertension?** | Atherosclerosis in late middle-aged and older persons and fibromuscular dysplasia in younger women |
| **What was the clinical clue that renovascular hypertension may be present in this patient?** | Precipitous rise in creatinine after initiation of ACE inhibitors |
| **How can it present?** | Refractory hypertension, hypertension with renal insufficiency, or renal insufficiency without hypertension (ischemic nephropathy) |
| **What risk factors does she have?** | Smoker, diabetes mellitus, older, long-standing essential hypertension |
| **What other risk factor might she have?** | Atherosclerotic disease |
| **What physical exam finding suggests the diagnosis?** | Abdominal upper quadrant bruit |
| **What is the workup for renovascular hypertension?** | Two major screening tests are renal artery duplex scan and captopril renogram. |
| **What are the major diagnostic tests?** | Renal angiography is the gold standard and, except in the most high probability cases, is most useful after obtaining an abnormal functional screening test. |
| **What other renal artery imaging tests are useful in defining renal artery anatomy?** | Magnetic resonance angiography, carbon dioxide angiography, and helical CT |
| **What is the treatment for renovascular hypertension?** | Medical therapy with lifestyle changes and drugs, renal angioplasty with stent placement or surgical revascularization |

## CONGESTIVE HEART FAILURE

CASE 7

*A 45-year-old female with history of urinary tract infections (UTIs), pyelonephritis, and tertiary syphilis presents to the clinic with insidious onset of dyspnea and heart palpitations. On physical examination, you are impressed by the rapid upstroke and downstroke of the pulse and appreciate a diastolic decrescendo murmur at the second intercostal space and a late diastolic rumble at the apex.*

| | |
|---|---|
| **What's your differential diagnosis?** | Aortic regurgitation, patent ductus arteriosus, pulmonary regurgitation |
| **What is most likely causing this murmur?** | Aortic regurgitation |
| **What is aortic regurgitation (AR)?** | Regurgitation of the blood flow back into the left ventricle due to a structural abnormality of the aortic valve, the ascending aorta, or both |
| **What risk factor does she have?** | History of tertiary syphilis |
| **What is the most common cause in** | |
|     **Adults?** | Bicusp aortic valve |
|     **Children?** | Congenitial ventricular septal defect with aortic valve prolapse |
| **What other causes are there?** | Infective endocarditis, myxomatous degeneration, aortic dissection, fenfluramine, dexfenfluramine, Takayasu's arteritis, and granulomatous arteritis |
| **Is her presentation consistent with AR?** | Yes. Dyspnea, palpitations, and orthopnea may all occur, but some patients are asymptomatic. |

| | |
|---|---|
| **Describe the murmur heard in AR on PE** | High-pitched diastolic decrescendo murmur at the left sternal border. There may be an apical diastolic rumble and/or an enlarged and displaced apical pulse. |

**Describe these PE exam findings:**

| | |
|---|---|
| **Quincke's pulse** | Visible pulsations in the capillaries with gentle compression of the nail bed |
| **Pulse pressure** | Widened pulse pressure (systolic BP elevated and diastolic BP <60 mm Hg) |
| **Corrigan's pulse** | Visualizing a "water-hammer pulse"—a rapid rise and sudden collapse of the pulse |
| **Traube's sign** | "Pistol-shot" sound heard over the femoral artery |
| **Austin Flint murmur** | Soft, low-pitched, rumbling mid-diastolic bruit caused by the displacement of the anterior leaflet of the mitral valve by the AR stream |

| | |
|---|---|
| **What tests should you order?** | Echocardiogram, chest x-ray, and EKG |

**Describe the result you expect on the**

| | |
|---|---|
| **EKG** | Usually normal, but may have findings of left ventricle hypertrophy (LVH) |
| **Chest x-ray** | Increased cardiothoracic ratio in chronic AR |
| **Echocardiogram?** | High-frequency diastolic fluttering of the anterior leaflet of the mitral valve from diastolic regurgitation from the aorta. Aortic valve findings differ based on etiology. |

| | |
|---|---|
| **How is it diagnosed?** | Physical examination and echocardiogram described above |

| | |
|---|---|
| **What is the treatment for AR?** | Avoid strenuous activity, antibiotic prophylaxis against endocarditis is advised, and vasodilator therapy |
| **What's the first choice for vasodilator therapy?** | ACE inhibitors |
| **What about second-line therapy?** | Hydralazine or nifedipine |
| **When is aortic valve replacement indicated?** | Heart failure despite medical therapy |

## CASE 8

*A 65-year-old male with history of BPH, hypertension, and hyperlipidemia presents to the clinic after having two near syncope events while climbing stairs at home and at a football stadium. During each episode he became severely dyspnic, resolving with rest. On physical exam you appreciate a dampened carotid upstroke, and late-peaking crescendo-decrescendo systolic ejection murmur at the left sternal boarder radiating to the carotid arteries.*

| | |
|---|---|
| **What's your differential diagnosis?** | Atypical angina, aortic stenosis, hypertrophic cardiomyopathy, mitral regurgitation, ventricular septal defect, and aortic sclerosis |
| **What is most likely?** | Aortic stenosis (AS) |
| **What is the classic presentation?** | Exertional dyspnea most common, followed by angina, syncope, and congestive heart failure (CHF) |
| **What causes these symptoms?** | Narrowing of the aortic valve orifice with progressive obstruction of left ventricular outflow leading to increased afterload leads to hypertrophy and wall stress resulting in decreased systemic and coronary blood flow |

**What are the causes of AS?**

Senile degenerative (most common, older patients, valve calcified and sclerosed), unicuspid or bicuspid valve (younger patients), rheumatic heart disease

**What are the findings of the physical examination?**

Dampened carotid upstroke, sustained left ventricular impulse, absent A2, and a late-peaking crescendo-decrescendo systolic ejection murmur at the left sternal boarder radiating to the carotid arteries

**What tests should you order?**

EKG, CXR, and echocardiogram

**What results do you expect on the**

**EKG?**

LVH with T-wave inversion

**CXR?**

Calcifications seen in the area of the aortic valve and often dilatation of the ascending aorta

**Echo?**

Left ventricular wall thickening with a narrowed aortic valve orifice, elevated aortic valve gradient

**How is it diagnosed?**

Characteristic physical examination with confirmation by echocardiography

**What is the treatment for mild AS?**

Avoid dehydration and vasodilatation (e.g., diuretics and nitrates). Antibiotic prophylaxis against endocarditis is required for dental procedures or surgery.

**Define severe AS**

Pressure gradient >50 mm Hg and valve area <1 cm$^2$

**What is the treatment of severe AS?**

Surgical valve replacement

**When is aortic valve replacement surgery indicated?**

Severe AS with symptoms (dyspnea, congestive heart failure, syncope, or angina)

## CASE 9

*A 28-year-old male returns to your clinic after complaining of worsening shortness of breath while playing soccer and a few episodes of passing out after getting out of a chair at his home. A brief physical exam reveals a sustained left ventricular apical impulse, S3, and a systolic ejection murmur.*

| | |
|---|---|
| **What diagnosis should you consider?** | Hypertrophic cardiomyopathy (HCM) |
| **What is HCM?** | Left and/or right ventricular hypertrophy, usually asymmetric, involving the intra-ventricular septum |
| **What are the causes?** | Often unknown, but an autosomal dominant hereditary form has been described |
| **Which symptoms suggest HCM?** | Triad of DOE, presyncope, and angina |
| **What is the range of presentations possible with HCM?** | Asymptomatic, any combination of classic trial above to sudden cardiac death |
| **What may be appreciated on physical examination by** | |
| **Palpation?** | Sustained left ventricular apex |
| **Auscultation?** | Harsh systolic ejection murmur with radiation to the base and apex (but not the neck) that increases with Valsalva maneuver or squat-to-stand maneuver and decreases with squatting and leg raising. S3 and S4 are both common. |
| **What EKG findings do you expect?** | LVH with deep, broad Q waves that simulate a myocardial infarction |
| **What are the associated CXR findings?** | Usually normal |
| **How is HCM diagnosed?** | Echocardiogram |

| | |
|---|---|
| **What is the treatment?** | Avoid competitive sports and strenuous activity. β-blockers. Consider implantable defibrillator (AICD) in patients at high risk for sudden death. |

## CASE 10

*A 38-year-old female with history of appendectomy, depression, and mitral valve prolapse presents to your clinic complaining of progressive fatigue and weakness over the last few months. She denies symptoms of depression and has been sleeping well despite waking up infrequently short of breath. On physical exam, you appreciate a holosystolic murmur with a diminished S1 and splitting of S2*

| | |
|---|---|
| **What's most likely causing her symptoms?** | Chronic mitral regurgitation |
| **What is mitral regurgitation (MR)?** | Reverse (regurgitant) blood flow across the mitral valve from the left ventricle (LV) into the left atrium |
| **What was her primary risk factor?** | Mitral valve prolapse |
| **Name some other risk factors.** | Rheumatic heart disease (1/3 of cases), mitral annular calcification (age-related), endocarditis, congenital, papillary muscle dysfunction (ischemia/myocardial infarction), and any disease that enlarges the left ventricle (cardiomyopathies) |
| **How does chronic MR classically present?** | Asymptomatic until late in the disease progression, then with fatigue and weakness followed by dyspnea, orthopnea, and paroxysmal nocturnal dyspnea |
| **How would acute MR commonly present?** | Dyspnea and pulmonary congestion, secondary to sudden increase in the left ventricular end-diastolic pressure and left atrial pressure in a normal left atrium and LV |

**What may be found on
      EKG?**

Left atrial enlargement or an LVH pattern. Atrial fibrillation may be present as the atrium enlarges.

**CXR?**

Straightening of the left heart border, an atrial double density, or elevation of the left main-stem bronchus. Mitral valve calcifications may be seen.

**What diagnostic test should you order?**

Echocardiogram

**What is the medical
treatment of MR?**

**Acute MR**

Intravenous vasodilators (nitroprusside), intravenous inotropes, and possibly intra-aortic balloon counterpulsation followed by mitral valve replacement

**Chronic MR**

Treat underlying cause (e.g., ischemia). Afterload reducing with ACE inhibitors is the initial treatment, considered for mitral valve replacement surgery.

## CASE 11

*A 62-year-old male with history of CAD s/p MI resulting in abnormal LV systolic function and CHF presents to the hospital after running out of his heart medications 3 days ago with gradual onset of dyspnea. It's so bad he can barely walk across the room and is unable to lie down without getting short-winded. He does not have any chest pain like he did before his last heart attack.*

**What is the most likely
cause of his dyspnea?**

Pulmonary edema from CHF secondary and noncompliance with medications

**What other causes should be
considered?**

Left ventricular failure, myocardial infarction, valvular heart disease, arrhythmias, and hypertensive crisis

**Why are patients with pulmonary edema short of breath (sob)?**

Congested lung tissue with fluid in the interstitial spaces and alveoli increases the diffusion gradient resulting in less oxygen transported to red blood cells.

**What symptoms are common with pulmonary edema?**

Dyspnea, tachypnea, anxiety, restlessness

**What physical exam findings of pulmonary edema should you look for?**

Rales, rhonchi, wheezing, use of accessory respiratory muscles. Pink frothy expectorate common in cardiogenic edema

**What labs and tests should be included in the workup?**

Chem 8, CXR, CBC, Ck-Mb, troponin, EKG, ABG

**What are the CXR findings?**

Diffuse bilateral interstitial and perihilar vascular engorgement, alveolar infiltrates

**What other CXR findings are more likely in cardiogenic edema?**

Kerley B lines, pleural effusions, possible enlarged heart

**Do the findings on CXR always correlate well with the clinical findings?**

No, it can take hours for CXR findings to appear once symptoms develop, and it may take days for the CXR to return to normal once therapy is initiated.

**How can cardiogenic and noncardiogenic edema be differentiated?**

Clinical history most often

**What is the treatment?**

Correct underlying cause, oxygen; diuretics (furosemide) in cardiogenic edema

**What lab value indicates adequate treatment?**

An arterial oxygen tension >60 mm Hg

**What additional pharmacologic agents may be used if above therapy is inadequate?**

Morphine sulfate, nitroglycerin, nitroprusside, and inotropic agents (e.g., dobutamine or phosphodiesterase inhibitors) can be helpful in cardiogenic edema.

| When is mechanical ventilation indicated? | Coexisting hypercapnia or inadequate oxygenation ($PaO_2$ <60 mm Hg on $FIO_2$ 100% by mask) |

## CHEST PAIN

### CASE 12

*A 34-year-old male heroin abuser returns to the ER again complaining of pain in triage thought to be fictitious in an effort to receive narcotics and is found to have a fever of 39°C, p95, bp 120/75, and r26. He describes sharp chest pain that worsens with deep breathing. It is not associated with exertion. He also complains of chills, dyspnea, and generalized weakness. Physical exam reveals a thin male with numerous skin popping sites on both forearms and legs, 3/6 systolic ejection murmur, normal breath sounds bilaterally, and splinter-like hemorrhages within the nail beds.*

| What infectious process can explain all this? | Infective endocarditis (IE) |
|---|---|
| What is it? | IE occurs when organisms colonize vegetations (nonbacterial thrombotic endocarditis) composed of fibrin and platelets which form in response to trauma to the endothelium or in areas of turbulent blood flow. |
| What is the pathogenesis of IE? | Transient bacteremia which occurs secondary to another infection or as a result of invasive procedures involving mucosal surfaces that are normally colonized with bacteria |
| What behavior in this patient most likely caused his bacteremia? | IVDA (unsterile needle and/or skin contamination) |
| What are the risk factors for persistent bacteremia and IE? | A previous episode of IE, mitral valve prolapse which is associated with mitral regurgitation, degenerative, calcific valvular disease, congenital cardiac |

disease (including patent ductus arteriosus, ventricular septal defect, aortic coarct, bicuspid aortic valve), rheumatic valvular disease, and prosthetic valves

**How does IE present?**

Patients may have an acute or subacute presentation. Common symptoms include fever, chills, weakness, dyspnea, sweats, anorexia, weight loss, malaise, myalgia/ arthalgia, headache, and stroke syndromes.

**What signs and symptoms are suggestive of right-sided IE in injection (IDUs)?**

IDUs present with similar systemic symptoms. In addition, they may have pleuritic chest pain due to septic pulmonary emboli to the lungs from right-sided (tricuspid valve) IE.

**What physical findings support the diagnosis of IE?**

Fever, heart murmur, splenomegaly, cutaneous lesions (petechiae, Osler's nodes, Janeway's lesions, splinter hemorrhages), retinal lesions (Roth's spots), clubbing, and focal neurologic findings if central nervous system embolic events have occurred

**How is the diagnosis of IE confirmed?**
    **Lab**

Blood cultures demonstrating persistent bacteremia

    **Imaging**

Echocardiography

**What test should be ordered if a transthoracic echocardiogram is negative for vegetations?**

Transesophageal echocardiogram (more sensitive)

**Which ECHO test is most sensitive?**

Transesophageal echocardiogram

**Does a negative echocardiogram by itself rule out infective endocarditis?**

No

**What blood culture results do you suspect in native valve IE in individuals who are not IDUs?**

**Most common**

Streptococci (mainly viridans strepto-cocci), staphylococci, and enterococci

**Less common**

Gram-negative organisms (including the members of the "HACEK" group—*Hemophilus, Actinobacillus, Cardiobacterium, Eikenella, and Kingella*) and fungi

**What is the most common cause of IE in IDUs?**

*Staphylococcus aureus*

**What is the most common cause of early (occurring within 60 days of surgery) prosthetic valve endocarditis?**

*Staphylococcus epidermidis.* Late PVE has a similar microbiology to native valve IE.

**How is IE treated?**

Antibiotics are given based on the identi-fication and susceptibilities of the infect-ing organisms.

**When is valve replacement warranted?**

Severe congestive heart failure, par-avalvular abscess, one or more major arterial embolic events, inability to steril-ize the blood cultures, or relapse after appropriate therapy

**When is antibiotic prophy-laxis recommended?**

Patients with known risk factor for IE who undergo procedures that are associ-ated with a risk of transient bacteremia

## CASE 13

*A 55-year-old previously healthy male presents to your office after recovering from a flu-like illness last week now complaining of persistent substernal non-radiating chest pain that worsens with inspiration and decreases when seated upright. It is not associated with exercise and the only thing that seemed to lessen the pain was over-the-counter ibuprofen.*

| | |
|---|---|
| **What diagnosis do you suspect?** | Acute pericarditis |
| **What are the symptoms of acute pericarditis?** | The one symptom is chest pain—usually substernal, constant, nonradiating; may worsen with inspiration, may lessen with sitting up. |
| **What are the most common pathogens in acute viral pericarditis?** | Echovirus and Coxsackie B5, B6 |
| **What drugs can cause pericarditis?** | Procainamide and hydralazine |
| **What are the physical signs of acute pericarditis?** | The one sign is the pericardial friction rub which may be present, absent, intermittent, or changing over time. |
| **What blood tests are specific for diagnosing acute viral pericarditis?** | None. Erythrocyte sedimentation rate will be increased and there may be a mild leukocytosis. |
| **What will be found on EKG?** | Diffuse ST segment elevations |
| **What's the treatment of acute viral pericarditis?** | Aspirin or a nonsteroidal anti-inflammatory drug |

## CASE 14

A 63-year-old male with history of uncontrolled hypertension secondary to noncompliance with medications presents after lifting heavy boxes in his basement with severe, sharp "tearing" sensation in the posterior chest and back followed by near syncope. EMS reported that his carotid pulsations were unequal and the blood pressure in his arms differed by >20 mm Hg.

| | |
|---|---|
| **What diagnosis do you suspect?** | Acute aortic dissection |
| **What else is in the differential?** | Pericarditis, pulmonary embolus, musculoskeletal pain, pleuritis, cholecystitis, peptic ulcer disease or perforating ulcer, acute pancreatitis |

| | |
|---|---|
| **Why do you suspect aortic dissection?** | Severe, sharp, or "tearing" posterior chest or back pain or anterior chest pain with or without radiation is characteristic. |
| **What additional features may be present?** | Syncope, a cerebrovascular accident, MI, or heart failure |
| **What's the pathophysiology behind aortic dissection?** | Blood separates the intima from the surrounding media and/or adventitia, creating a false lumen that produces pain |
| **What was his risk factor for a medial tear?** | Uncontrolled hypertension (most common) |
| **What other risk factors exist?** | Marfan's and Ehlers-Danlos syndromes, blunt chest trauma, bicuspid aortic valve, coarctation of the aorta, arteritis (especially giant cell), pregnancy (third trimester to several months postpartum), Noonan's and Turner's syndromes |
| **What may be found on physical exam?** | Weak or absent carotid, brachial, or femoral pulse resulting from the intimal flap or compression by hematoma |
| **What basic radiographic imaging test can be ordered to support the diagnosis?** | CXR revealing mediastinal and/or aortic widening |
| **What three things if present strongly support the diagnosis of aortic dissection?** | Acute onset of tearing and/or ripping chest pain, CXR revealing mediastinal and/or aortic widening, and unequal pulse pressure and/or blood pressure ($>20$ mm Hg difference between the right and left arms) |
| **Rank in descending order of sensitivity and specificity the imaging modalities for diagnosing aortic dissection.** | Magnetic resonance imaging, CT scan, contrast aortography, transesophageal echocardiography |
| **What is the medical treatment for acute aortic dissection?** | Antihypertensives ($\beta$-blocker, calcium channel blocker—verapamil or diltiazem) |

| | |
|---|---|
| **What additional blood pressure medication should be considered if blood pressure is unable to be controlled by one of the above medications?** | Infusion of vasodilator such as IV nitro-prusside |
| **What are the indications for surgical management of aortic dissection?** | Acute proximal dissection; acute distal dissection complicated by progression with vital organ compromise, rupture or impending rupture (saccular aneurysm formation), or retrograde extension into the ascending arch; any patient with Marfan's syndrome |

## CASE 15

*A 35-year-old male beginner snow-border presents to your office after returning from a ski trip out west where he complained of chest pain with movement. His father died of a heart attack and he is concerned he may be having an MI. The substernal chest pain does not occur with exertion like climbing stairs and he denies a history of diabetes, hyperlipidemia, or smoking. On physical exam, palpation over the sternum reproduces his pain.*

| | |
|---|---|
| **What's the diagnosis?** | Costochondral pain |
| **What symptoms are typical?** | Sharp localized pain in the anterior chest that is reproducible with palpation |
| **Where does the pain come from?** | Rib bones or rib cartilage |
| **What is the main risk factor?** | Recent chest trauma (e.g., falls, motor vehicle accident, etc.) |
| **How is it diagnosed?** | History, presentation with pain on palpation |
| **What is the treatment?** | NSAIDs |

CASE 16

*A 72-year-old male with history of hypertension, diabetes, hyperlipidemia, smoking, peripheral vascular disease s/p vascular bypass presents to your clinic complaining of fatigue and substernal chest discomfort for the last few weeks. He describes the chest pain as a band-like squeezing sensation that gradually comes on with exertion and is relieved with rest. On occasions the discomfort radiates down his left arm. The chest pain does not change with position or respiration. He came in today because the pain has not gone away for hours.*

| | |
|---|---|
| **What do you suspect?** | Acute myocardial infarction (AMI) |
| **What's the mechanism responsible for the vast majority of myocardial infarctions?** | Disruption of atherosclerotic plaque, leading to platelet aggregation, thrombus formation, and occlusion of an epicardial coronary artery |
| **How does AMI commonly present?** | Severe substernal pressure or pain with radiation to the left arm, back, or jaw |
| **What are his risk factors for AMI?** | Cigarette smoking, diabetes mellitus, hypertension, hypercholesterolemia |
| **Is family history important?** | Yes, history of CAD in a primary relative (parent, sibling, or offspring) is a risk factor as well |
| **What other potentially catastrophic conditions should be considered when considering AMI?** | Pulmonary embolus, dissecting thoracic aortic aneurysm |
| **What physical exam findings may be present in AMI?** | Pale, diaphoresis, cyanosis, weak pulse, distant heart sounds, S4 |
| **What finding on PE would suggest papillary muscle necrosis?** | Blowing systolic murmur |
| **What diagnostic labs and tests should be ordered?** | Creatine kinase (Ck)-MB, troponin, EKG |

**How is AMI diagnosed?**

Chest discomfort characteristic of ischemia with typical EKG changes and elevations in serum markers of myocardial injury (CK-MB and troponin)

**What are the minimum ST elevation criteria for diagnosing an acute myocardial infarction?**

ST elevation in two contiguous leads: 0.1 mV in the limb leads; 0.2 mV in the precordial leads; 0.05 mV in leads $RV_3$ and $RV_4$

**What single drug has been proven effective in both primary and secondary prevention of myocardial infarction?**

Aspirin

**What types of medication have been shown to improve long-term prognosis after an acute myocardial infarction?**

Aspirin, β-blockers, statins, and, in patients with reduced left ventricular ejection fraction, ACE inhibitors

**What is the treatment for acute ST segment elevation myocardial infarction?**

In the absence of contraindications, IV administration of a thrombolytic (also known as fibrinolytic) agent. In hospitals with a cardiac catheterization laboratory and cardiac surgery, primary percutaneous transluminal coronary angioplasty is an alternative treatment if it can be performed in a timely fashion.

**What is the most devastating complication of administering a thrombolytic agent?**

Both major and minor bleeding complications can occur. In 0.1% of cases an intracranial bleed occurs, resulting in a hemorrhaging stroke.

## CASE 17

*A 45-year-old male presents to your office after being discharged from the hospital 1 week ago for pneumonia complaining of worsening sob and cough with a sharp stabbing left-sided chest pain that worsens with inspiration. He says that he was unable to complete his course of antibiotics because he could not afford the co-pay.*

| | |
|---|---|
| **What's most likely causing his pain?** | Pleurisy |
| **How does it commonly present?** | Dyspnea with a sharp, stabbing, unilateral, pleuritic chest pain |
| **What is it?** | Inflammation of parietal pleura of the lungs |
| **What can cause it?** | Connective tissue disease, lung/chest wall abscess, and pneumonia |
| **What other common causes exist?** | Malignancy (bronchial carcinoma), pulmonary infarction, and pneumothorax |
| **What may be appreciated on physical exam?** | Restricted breathing on affected side and friction rub on auscultation |
| **What may the CXR reveal?** | Pleural effusion |
| **How is it diagnosed?** | History and presentation |
| **What is the treatment?** | Correct underlying cause (complete course of antibiotics), NSAIDs, and aspirin |

## CASE 18

*A 66-year-old male with history of HTN, CAD s/p MI and 2 vessel coronary artery bypass grafts (CABGs) 2 years ago presents to the ER after a MVC complaining of deep boring pain in the back that was not relieved by his prn sublingual nitroglycerin or ES Tylenol. The pain is not like his prior angina pain.*

| | |
|---|---|
| **What's your differential?** | MI, pancreatitis, vertebral fracture, AAA |
| **Physical exam reveals a pulsating mass in the abdomen. What diagnosis is number one in your differential now?** | Abdominal aortic aneursym (AAA) |

**Why?**

Patient has identifiable risk factors for AAA and findings on physical exam are consistent with the diagnosis.

**What are the risk factors?**

Atherosclerosis (most common), hypertension, smoking, family history of AAA, trauma, vasculitis, and Marfan's syndrome

**Is this patient's presentation typical?**

No. Patients often present asymptomatic, but may present with a deep boring pain in the low back or flank as in this patient.

**What's your best screening test?**

Ultrasound (to locate and determine size of AAA)

**Diagnostic test?**

CT with IV contrast

**CT confirms localized dilatation of the abdominal aorta. What determines your therapy?**

Centimeters of dilatation

**What's the therapy of an AAA at**
**<5 cm?**

Outpatient management with periodic ultrasounds to assess growth and current size

**>5 cm?**

Elective surgical resection of aneurysm and synthetic graft replacement

**Why perform surgery at >5 cm?**

Statistically significant risk of rupture

**How does a ruptured AAA present?**

Severe abdominal pain with hypotension, shock, or myocardial ischemia

**What's the treatment for a ruptured AAA?**

IV fluids, transfusion with packed RBCs as needed, and urgent surgery

## ARRHYTHMIAS AND CONDUCTION DISORDERS

### CASE 19

*A 63-year-old male with history of HTN presents to your clinic with complaints of palpitations on and off for the last 2 weeks. Physical exam reveals an irregular heart rhythm. EKG is shown (Fig. 1-1).*

| | |
|---|---|
| **What's the diagnosis?** | Atrial fibrillation (AF) |
| **Describe the diagnostic EKG findings.** | EKG showing irregular fluctuating baseline without any visible P waves with an irregular ventricular response |
| **Were his symptoms consistent with the diagnosis?** | Yes, palpitations is a common complaint. |
| **What other symptoms may patients present with?** | "Skipped" beats, light-headedness, breathlessness, angina, and syncope |
| **What was his risk factor?** | Hypertension |
| **What other risk factors should be considered?** | Drugs (cocaine, ethanol, theophylline, and caffeine), hyperthyroidism, pericarditis, ischemia, and MI |
| **What is the initial treatment in the setting of hemodynamic compromise (myocardial ischemia, MI, hypotension, or CHF)?** | Prompt electric cardioversion |

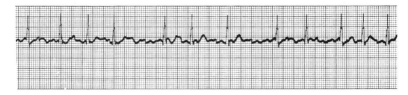

**Figure 1-1.**
*Source:* Smeltzer SC, Bare BG. Textbook of Medical-Surgical Nursing, 9th Ed. Philadelphia: Lippincott Williams & Wilkins, 2000.

| | |
|---|---|
| **What is the initial treatment goal in mild well-tolerated cases?** | Control ventricular rate with calcium channel blockers, β-blockers, or digoxin and correct underlying cause. |
| **When is digoxin use preferred?** | In patients with coexisting CHF or severe LV dysfunction |
| **What is the next therapy if AF has been present for greater than 48 hours at presentation?** | Anticoagulation for 3 weeks before and after cardioversion |
| **What purpose does anticoagulation serve?** | Decrease risk of thromboembolic event |
| **When is cardioversion without anticoagulation acceptable?** | If AF has been present for less than 48 hours at presentation |
| **What cardioversion therapy should be used first?** | Chemical cardioversion with quinidine or procainamide |
| **What alternative cardioversion therapy is available if pharmacotherapy fails?** | Electric cardioversion |

CASE 20

*A 72-year-old female presents with lightheadedness and pulse rate around 150 with the EKG shown (Fig. 1-2).*

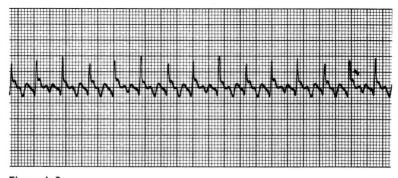

**Figure 1–2.**
*Source:* Nettina, SM. The Lippincott Manual of Nursing Practice, 7th Ed. Lippincott Williams & Wilkins, 2001.

**What's the diagnosis?**　　　　Atrial flutter

**How is it diagnosed?**　　　　EKG showing regular undulation (saw-
　　　　　　　　　　　　　　　tooth pattern) in the baseline with an
　　　　　　　　　　　　　　　atrial rate of 280–350

**What underlying causes**　　　Hypertension, drugs (cocaine, ethanol,
**should be looked for?**　　　　theophylline, and caffeine), hyperthy-
　　　　　　　　　　　　　　　roidism, pericarditis, ischemia, and MI

**What's the typical presenta-**　Usually asymptomatic, but may experi-
**tion?**　　　　　　　　　　　ence palpitations, syncope, and
　　　　　　　　　　　　　　　light-headedness with higher heart
　　　　　　　　　　　　　　　rates

**What is the treatment?**　　　Correct underlying cause and consider
　　　　　　　　　　　　　　　low-voltage synchronized electric car-
　　　　　　　　　　　　　　　dioversion if patient becomes unstable
　　　　　　　　　　　　　　　(e.g., hypotension, ischemic pain, or
　　　　　　　　　　　　　　　severe CHF)

## CASE 21

*A 44-year-old female presents complaining of infrequent heart palpitations
and occasional light-headness. On exam, you appreciate a pulse rate of 180.
The EKG is shown (Fig. 1-3).*

**What's the diagnosis?**　　　　AV nodal re-entrant tachycardia

**What is it?**　　　　　　　　　The most common paroxysmal supraven-
　　　　　　　　　　　　　　　tricular tachycardia that originates above
　　　　　　　　　　　　　　　the ventricles in the AV junction

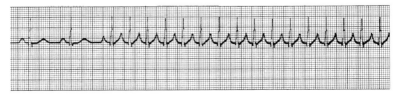

**Figure 1–3.**
*Source:* Smeltzer SC, Bare BG. Textbook of Medical-Surgical Nursing, 9th Ed. Philadelphia:
Lippincott Williams & Wilkins, 2000.

| | |
|---|---|
| **What EKG findings are diagnostic?** | Tachycardia and a characteristic pattern of P waves hidden in the T waves |
| **Was this presentation common?** | Yes, patients often present with sudden transient episodes of increased heart rate (150–250) with or without symptoms (palpitations, light-headedness, angina, and syncope). |
| **What can cause it?** | Stress, increased catecholamines, or MI |
| **What is the initial therapy?** | Vagal maneuvers (carotid sinus massage and Valsalva maneuver) |
| **What is the next step if vagal maneuvers fail?** | Adenosine, verapamil, or diltiazem to slow or block the AV node |

## CASE 22

*Your medical resident calls you to 5 North to witness a cardiac arrest. As you enter the room he hands you the EKG shown (Fig. 1-4).*

| | |
|---|---|
| **What's your diagnosis?** | Torsades de pointes (TdP) |
| **What is the diagnostic EKG pattern?** | A polymorphic ventricular tachycardia with QRS complexes that progressively change direction |

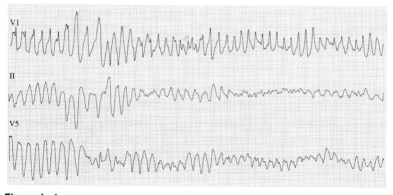

**Figure 1–4.**
*Source:* Wagner GS. Marriott's Practical Electrocardiography, 10th Ed. Philadelphia: Lippincott Williams & Wilkins, 2001.

**What is the main risk factor?**     A prolonged QT interval

**What can prolong the QT interval?**     Hypocalcemia, quinidine, and procainamide

**What is the treatment?**     IV bolus of magnesium sulfate and discontinue offending agents

**What is an alternative therapy to magnesium sulfate?**     Increase heart rate to 90–120 bpm using either isoproternol or temporary pacing (both treatments shorten the QT interval)

**When should electric cardioversion be considered?**     In cases of sustained TdP despite above measures

## CASE 23

*A 35-year-old male diagnosed with metastatic colon cancer undergoes aggressive experimental chemotherapy and is found unresponsive at home after his second course of therapy. He arrives by EMS with the EKG shown (Fig. 1-5).*

**What's the diagnosis?**     Ventricular fibrillation

**Define it.**     A cardiac arrhythmia characterized by uncoordinated ventricular depolarizations and contractions that can result in absence of cardiac output and rapid death

**Describe the diagnostic EKG findings.**     Undulating baseline with no identifiable P waves or QRS complexes

**What main risk factor should be considered?**     Recent severe acute MI

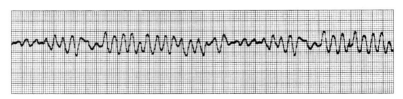

**Figure 1–5.**
*Source:* Smeltzer SC, Bare BG. Textbook of Medical-Surgical Nursing, 9th Ed. Philadelphia: Lippincott Williams & Wilkins, 2000.

**What is the treatment?**   Immediate unsynchronized electric cardioversion while giving epinephrine and then lidocaine

**What is the next step once patient is cardioverted?**   Continue lidocaine until any reversible causes can be corrected

## CASE 24

*A 52-year-old male complains of palpitations after watching his son's football team lose their opening game then passes out. Medical staff rushes to his side with an AED and the rhythm in Figure 1-6 shows up on the screen.*

**What's the diagnosis?**   Ventricular tachycardia

**Describe the diagnostic EKG findings.**   EKG showing a series of three or more successive ventricular contractions (PVCs) with a wide QRS (usually >120 ms) at a rate of 100–250 bpm

**What possible underlying causes are there?**   Ischemia (coronary artery disease), MI, electrolyte imbalance, drugs, and cardiomyopathy

**What is the treatment if patient is**
  **Clinically stable?**   Pharmacologic cardioversion with IV lidocaine (or procainamide) and correct underlying cause

  **Hemodynamically unstable?**   Synchronized electric cardioversion

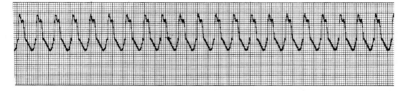

**Figure 1–6.**
*Source:* Smeltzer SC, Bare BG. Textbook of Medical-Surgical Nursing, 9th Ed. Philadelphia: Lippincott Williams & Wilkins, 2000.

# SHOCK

## CASE 25

*A 23-year-old male previously healthy presents to the ER by ambulance after being found in a parking lot with one anterior chest stab wound. Upon EMS arrival, the patient was alert and orientated, mildly tachycardic, and tachypnic with normal blood pressure. Physical exam revealed a 2-cm linear laceration just left of the sternum. En route to the ER EMS reports that his blood pressure is falling and jugular venous distention (JVD) is now evident on physical exam.*

| | |
|---|---|
| **What's your differential diagnosis for hypotension and JVD?** | Tension pneumothorax, cardiac tamponade, air embolism, and myocardial dysfunction |
| **Which two are more likely in this patient?** | Tension pneumothorax and cardiac tamponade |
| **On exam, his lung sounds are normal, but decreased heart sounds are appreciated. Which do you suspect now?** | Cardiac tamponade |
| **What is the most common cause of cardiac tamponade?** | Penetrating trauma to the anterior chest |
| **What are the causes of cardiac tamponade in the nontrauma patient?** | Metastatic malignancy (lung and breast most commonly), uremia, bacterial or tubercular pericarditis, anticoagulant hemorrhage, systemic lupus erythematosis, postradiation |
| **What is the mechanism behind cardiac tamponade?** | Accumulation of intrapericardial fluid causes an increase in intrapericardial pressure. When this pressure exceeds the right atrial (RA) filling pressure, there is a decrease in the amount of blood delivered to the ventricles. The resultant decreased stroke volume may lead to hemodynamic compromise. |

**What are the clinical features of cardiac tamponade?**

Classically, pulsus paradoxus >15 mm Hg, hypotension, JVD, and diminished heart sounds. Hypotension, JVD, and diminished heart sounds are known as Beck's triad.

**What is pulsus paradoxus?**

An abnormal drop in blood pressure during inspiration, due to the increase in afterload caused by negative intrapleural pressure

**What labs should you order?**

Comprehensive metabolic panel, complete blood count, pt, ptt, inr

**What other tests should you order?**

EKG, CXR, and trans-thoracic echocardiogram (TTE)

**What results to you expect to find on**
    **EKG?**

It may show low QRS voltage and T-wave flattening, and may demonstrate electrical alternans (beat-to-beat variation in P- and R-wave amplitude).

    **CXR?**

It may demonstrate a normal or enlarged cardiac silhouette, with clear lung fields.

    **TTE?**

It may demonstrate as little as 15 ml of intrapericardial fluid. It may also demonstrate RA compression and RV diastolic collapse.

**How is the diagnosis of cardiac tamponade made?**

Based on clinical findings

**What is the treatment of cardiac tamponade?**

Fluid resuscitation via two large bore peripheral IV lines, followed by pericardiocentesis and thoracotomy. Pericardiocentesis is both diagnostic and therapeutic, but thoracotomy is the definitive therapy.

CASE 26

*A 17-year-old female recently diagnosed with exudative pharyngitis presents to the ER with acute onset generalized rash, flushing, angioedema, headache, and near syncope after taking her first dose of her antibiotic. EMS reports her blood pressure is 90/50 with a pulse of 125.*

| | |
|---|---|
| **What do you suspect?** | Anaphylactic shock (AS) second to allergic reaction to penicillin |
| **Name other causes of shock.** | Cardiogenic, hemorrhagic, hypovolemic, septic |
| **What is anaphylaxis?** | An acute systemic reaction involving multiple organ systems to an IgE-mediated release of chemical mediators from mast cells and basophils, occurring in previously sensitized individuals, resulting in circulatory and respiratory collapse |
| **What most likely triggered her attack?** | PCN |
| **Name other causes of anaphylaxis.** | Bee stings, nuts, shellfish |
| **Name the major spontaneously generated vasoactive mediator that results in anaphylaxis.** | Arachidonic acid, leading to formation of leukotrienes, prostaglandins, thromboxane, prostacyclins |
| **Will any lab or imaging tests aid in making the diagnosis?** | No |
| **How is the diagnosis of AS made?** | Clinical history and physical exam |
| **What is the initial management of AS?** | Airway, breathing, circulation (ABCs) |
| **What is the management after the initial ABCs?** | Two large bore IV lines, fluid resuscitation, monitor, EPI, other pharmacological aids |

| | |
|---|---|
| **What pharmacological aids are used to counteract AS?** | Isotonic IV fluids, EPI, diphenhydramine, albuterol, solumedrol, aminophiline, glucagon, dopamine, cimetidine |

## CASE 27

*A 62-year-old female with known CAD s/p stent to right coronary artery 1 year ago presents to ER with 10/10 substernal pressure with radiation to neck and down right arm relieved partially by taking sublingual nitroglycerin at home. EMS reports that the patient has become more anxious and her skin has become cool and clammy while her heart rate increased.*

| | |
|---|---|
| **What is her initial symptom complex consistent with?** | Acute myocardial infarction (AMI) |
| **What complication do you suspect after hearing the EMS report?** | Cardiogenic shock second to AMI |
| **What are the clinical S/Sx of cardiogenic shock (CS)?** | Cool, clammy skin; oliguria; anxiety; confusion, tachycardia, increased vascular resistance |
| **What is CS?** | Hypoperfusion of tissues with failure to meet metabolic demand, and systolic blood pressure (SBP) <90 mm Hg, caused by inadequate myocardial contractility or by mechanical impairment of the heart |
| **What is the incidence of CS after an AMI?** | 5–7% |
| **What are some of the independent predictors of risk for developing CS post-AMI?** | Advanced age, female, large or anterior wall MI, previous MI, history of CHF, multivessel coronary artery disease, proximal occlusion of the left anterior descending artery, and diabetes mellitus |
| **What is the predominant cause of CS?** | LV infarction |

| | |
|---|---|
| **What mechanical impairments can lead to CS?** | Pericardial tamponade, massive pulmonary embolism (PE), acute mitral valve insufficiency, aortic dissection, ventricular septal wall rupture |
| **In addition to an AMI, what other etiologies of decreased myocardial contractility can lead to CS?** | Myocardial contusion, toxins or drugs, cardiomyopathy, dysrhythmias, heart block |
| **What blood pressure parameters are more sensitive measures of shock than SBP?** | Mean arterial pressure (MAP): decrease >30 mm Hg; pulse pressure: <20 mm Hg |
| **What lab studies are ordered to assess CS?** | Arterial blood gas, serum bicarbonate or lactate, CK, CK-MB, and troponin |
| **What additional tests should you order?** | CXR, EKG, and transthoracic echo |
| **What are the initial steps for stabilization of CS?** | Oxygen, IV access, cardiac monitor, continuous pulse oximetry |
| **What is the first drug given in the setting of an AMI?** | Aspirin, 325 mg orally |
| **What is the first-line treatment for RV infarction with hypotension?** | Rapid IV infusion of 1 liter 0.9 normal saline (NS), followed by dobutamine if no response |
| **What drug increases myocardial contractility and augments coronary blood flow but does not induce reflex tachycardia?** | Dobutamine |
| **What drug is used in the setting of profound hypotension?** | Dopamine |
| **If shock persists after using drugs, what do you use?** | Intraortic balloon pump |

## CASE 28

*A 62-year-old White male with history of smoking, hypertension, and psoriasis develops progressive abdominal pain and light-headness prior to EMS arriving. EMS finds tachycardia, tachypnea, cool clammy skin with poor capillary refill, pulsatile abdominal mass, and a systolic blood pressure of 72 mm Hg. His friend said before this happened he felt his heart beating in his abdomen.*

| | |
|---|---|
| **The SBP of 72 mm Hg is consistent with what diagnosis?** | Shock |
| **What types of shock are there?** | Cardiogenic, hemorrhagic, hypovolemic, septic, and anaphylactic |
| **What type do you suspect here?** | Hemorrhagic |
| **What is hemorrhagic shock?** | Tissue hypoxemia and hypoperfusion caused by rapid blood loss of sufficient quantity to overcome the body's compensatory mechanisms |
| **What are the classic signs of acute hemorrhage?** | Tachycardia, tachypnea, narrow pulse pressure, cool and clammy skin, oliguria, low central venous pressure (CVP), altered mental status, hypotension |
| **What are the 4 major etiological sources of acute hemorrhage?** | Trauma, gastrointestinal tract, reproductive tract, vascular |
| **Do his complaints of abdominal pain with a pulsating sensation help you determine a possible cause?** | Yes, abdominal and/or back pain with a pulsating character is consistent with AAA. |
| **What are his risk factors for AAA?** | Hypertension, White, male, smoking, age |
| **What other risk factors exist?** | Atherosclerosis and family history |
| **What is the initial management of hemorrhagic shock?** | Airway, breathing, circulation (ABCs) |

**What is the management after the initial ABCs?**

Two large bore IV lines; fluid resuscitation; monitor

**In restoring circulation, why is the preferred route of venous access two large bore (16-gauge preferred) peripheral IV lines?**

Peripheral IVs instill fluids faster secondary to their short length and larger diameter

**List the basic methods of hemodynamic monitoring for shock.**

Electrocardiogram; pulse oximeter; CVP; end tidal carbon dioxide; arterial blood pressure, pulse, pulse pressure, respiratory rate

**Name the resuscitation fluid of choice for the initial management of hemorrhagic shock.**

0.9 NS or Ringers lactate

**When giving a fluid challenge, what is the optimal body position?**

Supine, with legs elevated

**What STAT labs should you order?**

CBC, CMP, coags, type and cross for 6 PRBC

**What imaging test will confirm your diagnosis?**

Abdominal ultrasound

**What STAT consult should you order?**

Vascular surgery

**What physiological indices can you use to gauge your resuscitation efforts?**

Heart rate, blood pressure, capillary refill, urine output, CVP

**After 0.9 NS, what natural colloid should be used next for fluid resuscitation?**

Packed red blood cells

**What is the survival rate of patients who experience a ruptured abdominal aortic aneurysm?**

Less than 50%

## CASE 29

*An 88-year-old nursing home patient with history of scleroderma and severe reflux disease with recurrent aspiration, urinary incontinence second to prostate cancer surgery years ago, and prior UTIs is transferred to the ER from his nursing home after becoming disorientated and hypotensive. Upon arrival, he is alert, but disorientated. Temperature is 38.5°C, pulse 110, blood pressure 85/60 with a respiratory rate of 25.*

| | |
|---|---|
| **What diagnosis is likely based on his vital signs?** | Shock |
| **What is the differential for shock?** | Cardiogenic, hemorrhagic, hypovolemic, septic, and anaphylactic |
| **Which is more likely here?** | Septic shock |
| **What vital sign tipped you off?** | Temp >38°C |
| **What are the 3 major organ sources of sepsis?** | Abdomen, lungs, urinary tract |
| **What other organ systems should be focused on?** | CNS, skin, and soft tissue |
| **Which organ sources are most likely in this patient?** | Lung and urinary tract |
| **What risk factors does this patient have for lung and urinary infection?** | Dysphagia with aspiration risk (pneumonia risk) and urinary incontinence with prior UTIs |
| **What's required to diagnose sepsis?** | At least two of the following: 1) temperature >38°C or <36°C; 2) heart rate >90 beats per minute; 3) respiratory rate >20 breaths per minute or $PaCO_2$ <32 mm Hg; 4) white blood count >12,000/$\mu$L, <4,000/$\mu$L, or >10% bands |
| **Are the criteria met?** | Yes |

| | |
|---|---|
| **What is the first priority in the management of septic shock?** | ABCs |
| **What is the management after the initial ABCs?** | Two large bore IV lines, fluid resuscitation, monitor heart rate and blood pressure for response |
| **What stat labs should you order?** | CBC with differential, CMP, PT/INR, UA, UCX, blood cultures x2, sputum Gram-stain culture and sensitivity, CK-MB, troponin |
| **What imaging should you order?** | CXR |
| **What cardiac test should you order?** | EKG |
| **What type of medication is critical in septic shock?** | Antibiotics |
| **What guides your choice of antibiotic therapy?** | Empiric coverage for Gram-negative and Gram-positive bacteria. Coverage should be adjusted later once organism is identified and drug sensitivities are known. |

## MISCELLANEOUS DISORDERS

### CASE 30

A 58-year-old female with history of CVA, diabetes, and HTN presents with infrequent calf pain after walking roughly 2 blocks that abates after slowing down or stopping.

| | |
|---|---|
| **What diagnosis do you suspect?** | Claudication |
| **Why?** | Because it often presents with intermittent pain in an extremity with exercise or exertion and is relieved with rest. |

**What causes it?**

Peripheral arterial vascular insufficiency in the extremities

**What risk factors does this patient have for it?**

Atherosclerosis and an atherosclerotic event (e.g., stroke, MI), diabetes

**What other risk factors may other patients have?**

Thrombosis, embolism, or trauma

**What "classic" physical exam findings will you look for?**

5 Ps: pain, pallor, pulselessness, paresthesia, and paralysis (end stage)

**What additional finding may be found on physical exam?**

Cool skin, hair loss, ulceration, and muscle atrophy in the affected area

**What basic bedside test can support the diagnosis of claudication?**

Ankle-brachial index (ABI) to assess vascular insufficiency

**How do you calculate the ABI?**

Ratio of systolic blood pressure (SBP) in the ankle to the SBP in the arm

**What do the following results suggest?**
    **ABI <1**

Mild PVD

    **ABI <0.5**

Severe PVD

**ABI is 0.8. What additional tests will confirm your diagnosis?**

Ultrasound of affected area (assess vascular patency) and angiography (confirm ultrasound findings)

**Imaging confirms mild disease. What's the treatment?**

Diet, daily walking (increases collateral circulation), stop smoking, and reassess diabetic therapy if diabetes is present

**What if the severe disease (ABI <0.5) with rest pain was present?**

Surgical revascularization with autologous or synthetic grafting

# 2 Pulmonary Disorders

## INFECTIOUS DISEASES

### CASE I

*A 54-year-old male with history of diabetes, chronic obstructive pulmonary disease (COPD), peptic ulcer disease (PUD), hypertension (HTN), and degenerative joint disease (DJD) presents to your clinic complaining of sudden onset of fever, productive cough with brown colored sputum, dyspnea on exertion, and right lateral chest pain. His temperature is 103°F, pulse of 88, and respiratory rate of 26.*

| | |
|---|---|
| **What diagnosis are you considering?** | Community-acquired pneumonia (CAP) |
| **What were the clues?** | Sudden onset of fever, cough productive of purulent sputum, shortness of breath with or without pleuritic chest pain |
| **Is this patient's presentation characteristic of typical or atypical pneumonia?** | Typical |
| **How might atypical pneumonia present?** | Gradual onset of dry cough, fevers, prominent extrapulmonary symptoms such as headaches, myalgias, sore throat, nausea, vomiting, and diarrhea |
| **What are the most common organisms that cause "typical" CAP?** | *Streptococcus pneumoniae* and *Hemophilus influenzae* |
| **What are the most common organisms that cause "atypical" CAP?** | *Mycoplasma pneumoniae, Chlamydia* species, *Legionella pneumophilus*, influenza |
| **What risk factor does he have for pneumonia?** | COPD |

**What organisms are common in patients with pneumonia and COPD?**

*H. influenzae, S. pneumoniae, Legionella*

**Of these three organisms, which do you suspect this patient has?**

*S. pneumoniae* because he described his sputum as brown which can be implied to mean rust colored

**What organism would you have suspected if he had HIV?**

*Pneumocystis carinii*

**Recent seizures?**

Aspiration pneumonia with mouth flora (*Peptostreptococcus, Fusobacterium, Bacteroides melaninogenicus,* aerobic streptococci)

**Alcoholism?**

*Klebsiella, S. pneumoniae, H. influenzae*

**What finding on your lung exam would support pneumonia?**

Localized rales or evidence of consolidation

**What's your basic diagnostic workup?**

Chem 8 (important to assess renal function if planning on giving antibiotics), complete blood cell count (CBC) with differential (looking for evidence of infection) and sputum Gram stain and culture (attempt to identify organism), chest x-ray (CXR), arterial blood gas (ABG) if severely dyspneic, blood cultures if hospitalized

**What results do you expect in this patient with suspected CAP?**

**CBC**

Leukocytosis with a left shift (increased pneutrophils)

**CXR**

Right lower lobe (RLL) infiltrate (patient complained of right-sided pleuritic pain)

| | |
|---|---|
| **CXR reveals RLL infiltrate consistent with pneumonia, CBC positive for leukocytosis of 15,000 with left shift. What's your treatment plan?** | Empiric therapy with a macrolide (e.g., erythromycin, azithromycin) or a fluoroquinolone (e.g., levofloxacin) |

CASE 2

*A 66-year-old male with history of autoimmune hepatitis (recently prescribed azathioprine in addition to prednisone), hyperlipidemia, diabetes, and end-stage renal disease on hemodialysis is observed to be coughing blood-streaked phlegm while being hooked up to the dialysis equipment. The dialysis nurse further informs you that the patient is febrile at 103°F.*

| | |
|---|---|
| **What differential are you considering?** | Neoplasm (primary or metastatic), pneumonia, bronchiectasis, tuberculosis (TB), vasculitis, anticoagulant drugs |
| **Which are you most concerned about?** | TB |
| **Why?** | Productive cough (often with blood streaking) associated with fevers/night sweats, malaise, anorexia, and weight loss are consistent with TB patients on presentation. |
| **What risk factors does he have for TB?** | Immunosuppressed with prednisone and immuran, >65 years old, diabetic, dialysis patient |
| **Which social groups are at high risk for TB?** | Immigrants from countries with high infection rates, residents of long-term care facilities, medically underserved |
| **What causes TB and how is it transmitted?** | *Mycobacterium tuberculosis.* Transmitted through respiratory droplets. |
| **What's your first order to the nurse?** | Isolate the patient in a negative pressure room; patient and staff must wear masks. |

**What tests should be performed?**

Sputum sample for acid fast bacilli (AFB) stain and mycobacterial culture, purified protein derivative (PPD) placement, labs, and CXR

**What labs and imaging should you order in the meantime?**

Chemistry panel, CBC with differential, liver chemistry tests, Prothrombin time (PT) and International normalized ratio (INR), CXR

**CXR reveals apical and posterior segment infiltrates with cavitation. What does this suggest?**

Reactivation TB

**What is often found in primary TB?**

Mid to lower lung zones infiltrate with or without cavitation

**Two days later you read the amount of induration on the PPD test and it is 12 mm. What does this indicate?**

TB infection

**How much induration is needed for a positive PPD in the following groups?**
    **High risk (HIV, close contact)**

$\geq$5 mm

    **Moderate risk (high risk medical condition, immigrants, health care workers)**

$\geq$10 mm Hg

    **Low risk (all others)?**

$\geq$15 mm

**What additional test can be performed if the diagnosis is not clear?**

Bronchoscopy with bronchoalveolar lavage and biopsy if sputum negative but high degree of suspicion

**What is the classic pathologic feature of TB?**

Caseating granuloma

| | |
|---|---|
| **Which groups always need prophylactic therapy for a positive PPD?** | Close contacts, HIV, recent infection, high-risk medical groups, health care workers |
| **Which groups need prophylaxis if <35 years** | Immigrants from high-risk areas, medically underserved, residents of long-term care facilities |
| **Which antibiotic is usually used for prophylaxis?** | Isoniazid |
| **What are the 2 major treatment principles for TB?** | Never treat with less than 2 drugs. Prolonged therapy is standard. |
| **What are the 2 standard treatment regimens for TB?** | Isoniazid, rifampin, and pyrazinamide for 2 months followed by isoniazid and rifampin for 4 months or isoniazid and rifampin for 9 months |
| **What is the standard regimen for drug-resistant TB?** | Initially add 12 additional antibiotics to the above 3 drugs (usually ethambutol or streptomycin). Drug regimen tailored after susceptibility testing available. |
| **What are common side effects of isoniazid?** | Hepatitis and peripheral neuropathy |
| **What drug can be given to prevent the peripheral neuropathy?** | Pyridoxine |

## OBSTRUCTIVE AND RESTRICTIVE DISEASES

CASE 3

*A 16-year-old previously healthy female presents to your office complaining of a few instances of difficulty breathing, dry cough, and wheezing that lasts less than an hour. She also notes some chest tightness. The symptoms occur more frequently when unloading boxes in the basement in their new home or picking fruit on the family farm.*

**What's your differential for a young child wheezing?**

Asthma, foreign body aspiration, cystic fibrosis, and viral bronchiolitis

**What diagnosis do you suspect in this child?**

Asthma

**Why?**

Intermittent episodes of shortness of breath, cough, and chest tightness are characteristic of asthma.

**What do you suspect is causing her asthma?**

Allergens at the farm (pollen) and basement (dust)

**What other asthma triggers might be presented to you?**

Irritants (fumes, smoke), chronic sinusitis, viral infection, exercise, cold weather, gastroesophageal reflux disease, and possibly aspirin (especially in patients with nasal polyps)

**What's the basic mechanism behind asthma?**

A reversible airways disease characterized by hyperresponsiveness and bronchoconstriction of the airways to specific and nonspecific stimuli

**What physical exam signs are present in mild attacks?**

Tachypnea, wheezing, and a prolonged expiratory phase

**What additional signs present in more severe attacks?**

Inability to speak more than a few words, accessory muscle use, pulsus paradoxus, and distant breath sounds

**In most cases, how is the diagnosis made?**

By history and response to bronchodilator during an attack because most patients are asymptomatic in the clinic

**What diagnostic test can you order to confirm obstructive lung disease when disease is active?**

Pulmonary function tests (PFT)

**What ratio and value signifies obstruction?**

FEV1/FVC ratio $<70\%$

| | |
|---|---|
| **What test can be performed if obstruction is not present on PFTs?** | Methacholine challenge test. A positive test supports the diagnosis of asthma while a negative test rules it out. |
| **What determines treatment?** | Frequency of symptoms |

**Define the following and specify appropriate treatment:**

| | |
|---|---|
| **Mild intermittent** | Less than 2 times a week; short-acting inhaled β-agonist as needed |
| **Mild persistent** | Greater than 2 times a week, less than daily; daily low-dose inhaled corticosteroids and short-acting β-agonist as needed |
| **Moderate persistent** | Daily symptoms or daily use of short-acting inhaled β-agonist; moderate-dose inhaled corticosteroids and long-acting β-agonist with short-acting β-agonist as needed |
| **Severe persistent** | Frequent symptoms with limited physical activity; high-dose inhaled corticosteroids, long-acting β-agonist, short-acting β-agonist, consider oral steroid |
| **What other measures are important in asthma treatment?** | Patient education, pollen/dust control, avoidance of triggers. Treat associated conditions, especially sinusitis and gastroesophageal reflux disease (GERD). |

## CASE 4

*A 45-year-old male construction worker with a history of hypertension, alcoholism, and chronic pancreatitis has been complaining of feeling short-winded over the last year and a half with wheezing and nonproductive hacking cough. It does not occur at any specific place or time and is not associated with substernal chest pain. A friend at the job site has been letting him use some inhaler which has helped during working hours, but symptoms return by the next morning.*

**What disease do you suspect?**

Chronic obstructive lung disease

**What major risk factor for COPD does he have?**

Tobacco smoking (90% of cases) and male gender

**What other risk factors are there?**

$\alpha$1-antitrypsin (AAT) deficiency, family history, Caucasian ethnicity, and lower socioeconomic status

**When should you suspect AAT disease?**

When COPD occurs in a nonsmoker

**Which 2 types of COPD are there?**

Chronic bronchitis and emphysema

**Which does he most likely have?**

Emphysema, due to lack of productive cough

**Define chronic bronchitis**

Chronic productive cough for 3 months in each of 2 consecutive years after other causes of chronic cough have been excluded (a clinical diagnosis)

**Define emphysema.**

Abnormal permanent enlargement of the airspaces distal to the terminal bronchioles, accompanied by destruction of their walls and without fibrosis (a pathologic diagnosis)

**What are common PE findings in**
    **Mild disease?**

Barrel chest, hyperresonant lungs, decreased breath sounds, prolonged expiration, distant heart sounds, wheezes

    **Severe disease?**

Cachexia, pursed lip breathing, accessory muscle use, cyanosis, accentuated P2 heart sound, and peripheral edema

**What basic tests should be included in the initial workup?**

CXR and PFT

| | |
|---|---|
| **What are the associated CXR findings in COPD?** | Low and flat diaphragms, bullae, increased retrosternal lucency, narrow heart shadow, and attenuation of lung markings; prominence of hilae and right ventricle in pulmonary hypertension |
| **What are the associated pulmonary function test findings?** | Reduced $FEV_1/FVC$, elevated total lung and functional residual capacities, increased residual volume, reduced diffusion capacity. Bronchodilator responsiveness is seen in 30%. |
| **When would you consider ordering a CT scan?** | Concern for underlying lung cancer second to strong smoking history or trying to characterize type of emphysema |
| **Which type of emphysema on CT is more common in smokers?** | Centrilobular emphysema which begins in the respiratory bronchioles, spreads peripherally, and involves upper lobes |
| **Which type of emphysema on CT is more common with AAT deficiency?** | Panacinar emphysema which involves the entire alveolus, and predominates in lower lobes |
| **What's the treatment?** | Smoking cessation counseling, ipratropium (an anticholinergic agent), and sympathomimetic β-2 agonists (e.g., albuterol, salmeterol) |
| **What preventive measures are important in COPD?** | Pneumococcal vaccine and yearly influenza vaccinations |
| **When is supplemental oxygen therapy warranted?** | Hypoxemic patients (improves dyspnea and survival) |
| **What additional treatment options exist if deficient in α1-antitrypsin?** | AAT supplementation |

## CASE 5

*A 47-year-old male is referred to your clinic after being worked up by his primary care physician for slowly progressive dyspnea over the last year with a nonproductive cough. He has been ruled out for common disorders such as asthma, COPD, heart failure, and psychiatric disease as possible causes. The referring doctor also completed an extensive workup for causes of interstitial lung disease such as sarcoidosis, occupational exposure, infection, radiation, drugs, and collagen vascular diseases and came up negative. The primary doctor suspects he may have idiopathic pulmonary fibrosis (IPF).*

| | |
|---|---|
| **What is interstitial lung disease?** | A heterogenous group of lung diseases characterized by inflammation and fibrosis of the interalveolar septum |
| **Why does the doctor suspect IPF?** | A middle-aged patient with insidious onset of dyspnea on exertion with a persistent nonproductive cough is characteristic of IPF. |
| **What's your first step in the workup?** | Confirm by history, physical exam, and review of the medical record that sarcoidosis, occupational exposure, infection, radiation, drugs, and collagen vascular diseases are unlikely causes of his presumed interstitial lung disease. |
| **What signs on physical exam support the diagnosis of interstitial lung disease?** | Bibasilar end-inspiratory (velcro-like) crackles and clubbing of the digits |
| **What tests should be ordered in the workup of IPF?** | ABG, PFT, CXR followed by CT of chest |
| **What are the associated findings on** | |
| **ABG?** | Mild respiratory alkalosis with a normal or reduced $PO_2$ |
| **PFT?** | Restrictive pattern, reduced lung compliance, and decreased DLCO |
| **CXR and thoracic CT scan?** | Diffuse bilateral reticular infiltrates, predominantly at bases; honeycombing in end-stage disease |

| | |
|---|---|
| **What procedure should confirm the diagnosis?** | Bronchoscopy with transbronchial biopsy to rule out more common disorders (i.e., sarcoidosis); ppen-lung biopsy for definitive diagnosis |
| **What are the treatment options for IPF?** | Corticosteroids, cytotoxic therapy (cyclophosphamide or azathioprine) followed by lung transplant if medical therapy fails |

## CASE 6

A 55-year-old recently retired male with history of arthritis secondary to being overworked at the maintenance department at an old steel factory comes to your office for the first time after his insurance was changed. His medical charts from his prior MD were faxed and included recent comprehensive blood work, screening colonoscopy, prostate-specific antigen (PSA), and stress test. The patient said the stress test, which was normal, was done for a workup of gradual onset of shortness of breath and a nonproductive cough over the last few years. His last doctor did not suspect lung disease as he has been a nonsmoker.

| | |
|---|---|
| **What do you suspect?** | Interstitial lung disease (ILD) |
| **What are the causes?** | Idiopathic (a diagnosis of exclusion), sarcoidosis, occupational exposure, infection, radiation, drugs, collagen vascular diseases |
| **Which do you suspect in this patient?** | Occupational exposure to inorganic dusts at work |
| **Why?** | Insidious onset of dyspnea and nonproductive cough, usually >20–25 years after occupational exposure, is consistent with the diagnosis. |
| **What inorganic dusts could he have been exposed to?** | Asbestos (steel workers), silica (sandblasting) |

| | |
|---|---|
| **What other inorganic dust exposure is less likely in his case?** | Coal dust (coal miners) |
| **What findings on physical exam would support the diagnosis of ILD?** | Bibasilar end-inspiratory (velcro-like) crackles and clubbing of the digits |
| **Are routine lab tests helpful in making a diagnosis?** | No, they are often nonspecific and unhelpful |
| **What basic lung function test is helpful?** | PFT |
| **What findings do you expect?** | Restrictive pattern with reduced lung compliance, and decreased DLCO |
| **Is a CXR helpful?** | Yes. It may reveal a radiographic pattern consistent with either asbestosis or silicosis. |
| **What CXR findings are associated with** | |
| **Asbestosis?** | Diffuse linear opacities in lower lung fields, pleural plaques, pleural effusions |
| **Silicosis?** | Multiple small nodules (usually upper lobe) and calcification of the hilar lymph nodes |
| **How is the diagnosis often made in ILD secondary to asbestosis or silicosis?** | History of exposure, radiographic findings, and exclusion of other causes |
| **What additional invasive procedure may be useful in diagnosing asbestosis?** | Bronchoscopic identification of asbestos fibers or bodies in BAL fluid or in biopsy tissue specimens with histologic evidence of fibrosis |
| **Is it required to make the diagnosis?** | No |

**What is the treatment of inorganic dust ILD secondary to asbestosis and silicosis?**

Prevention of infections (influenza, pneumococcal vaccines), smoking cessation, oxygen when needed

**What infection is associated with silicosis?**

Tuberculosis

## CASE 7

*A 66-year-old previously healthy male recently retired from the military after a thorough physical examination, screening lab tests, and procedures appropriate for his age. Since retiring, he has been helping his brother at his newly purchased farm. But recently he has been unable to help because by midday, after arriving early in the morning, he feels febrile, gets short of breath, and has a persistent cough. Each day for the last week his symptoms recur, but clear by the time he wakes up at his home the next morning.*

**What is his presentation consistent with?**

A form of organic dust exposure causing a form of ILD (a.k.a., hypersensitivity pneumonitis)

**What are two common occupations associated with organic dusts that cause ILD?**

Farming (thermophilic actinomyces, fungal species) and bird breeding (avian proteins)

**How does organic dust ILD (or hypersensitivity pneumonitis) present?**

Acute onset of fever, cough, dyspnea 3–6 hours after inhaling dust with improvement in 24 hours if no repeated exposure. Can progress to chronic dyspnea, and fatigue with repeated dust exposure.

**What CXR findings are associated with hypersensitivity pneumonitis?**

Interstitial and alveolar infiltrates, predominantly lower lobes, often fleeting. Fibrosis and honeycombing in chronic disease.

**How is the diagnosis made?**

Careful occupational or hobby history in a patient with ILD. Symptom-free periods outside of job/hobby suggest hypersensitivity pneumonitis.

| What is the treatment of hypersensitivity pneumonitis? | Avoid exposures to the offending dust; use of steroids in chronic disease |
|---|---|

## MISCELLANEOUS DISORDERS

### CASE 8

*A 45-year-old male with unknown medical history presents to the ER by ambulance after being found with labored breathing on the street. EMS informs you that his airway is patent, respirations have decreased to 25 after being administered supplemental oxygen, remaining vital signs are normal, and EKG is normal. The cardiology fellow has already evaluated patient and informs you that it's not his heart.*

| After examining the patient, what 2 lab tests will be helpful in determining the cause? | ABG (assess for hypoxic or hypercapnic state) and CXR |
|---|---|
| What's the diagnosis if $PaO_2$ is <55 mm Hg? | Hypoxemic respiratory failure |
| What about if $PaCO_2$ >45 mm Hg? | Hypercapnic respiratory failure |
| What's your differential for hypoxemic respiratory failure? | Pneumonia, acute respiratory distress syndrome (ARDS), congestive heart failure |
| What's your differential for hypercapnic failure? | Drug overdose (particularly narcotics, benzodiazepines), stroke, asthma, COPD exacerbations, amyotrophic lateral sclerosis, myasthenia gravis, disorders of the muscles (muscular dystrophy) |
| What is the treatment? | Establish and maintain patent airway, administer supplemental oxygen, maintain adequate alveolar ventilation, and treat underlying cause |

## CASE 9

*A 68-year-old male with history of hypertension, hyperlipidemia, and CAD admitted with a non-ST elevation myocardial infarction (MI) 4 days ago, status post urgent coronary artery bypass graft (CABG) after heart catherization revealed significant 2-vessel CAD, develops profound respiratory distress with oxygen desaturation requiring intubation after enteral tube feed was started to maintain his caloric requirements.*

| | |
|---|---|
| **What's your differential diagnosis?** | Pulmonary edema secondary to transient myocardial ischemia or cardiomyopathy, mitral valve rupture, alveolar hemorrhage, and ARDS |
| **What STAT labs and tests would be useful?** | Chem 8, CBC, ABG, CXR, EKG, and echocardiogram |
| **Results are as follows: ABG, acute respiratory alkalosis with low oxygen and carbon dioxide; CXR, diffuse bilateral alveolar infiltrates; EKG and echo, no change from prior studies. What's the most likely diagnosis?** | ARDS |
| **What are common causes of ARDS?** | Sepsis, aspiration of gastric content, pneumonia, and trauma with burns or shock requiring multiple transfusions |
| **What is the mechanism of ARDS?** | Vascular injury and cytokine release |
| **What is the treatment of ARDS?** | Supportive care (mechanical ventilation with PEEP to maintain adequate oxygenation, nutritional support, avoidance of nosocomial infection, antibiotics when indicated, low IVF to decrease risk of pulmonary edema) |

## CASE 10

*A 44-year-old male presents to your office with complaints of coughing up a few cups of blood over the last week. On exam, you are impressed by his cachectic appearance, alcohol on his breath, and pack of cigarettes rolled up in his sleeve. Otherwise, his vital signs and heart and lung exams appear normal.*

| | |
|---|---|
| **What is this patient's problem?** | Hemoptysis |
| **Is it massive?** | No, that would be 600 mL of blood in 24 hours or by unstable vital signs. |
| **What are the most common causes of hemoptysis?** | Bronchitis, bronchiectasis, lung cancer, pneumonia, tuberculosis, aspergilloma, lung abscesses, septic emboli |
| **What do you suspect this patient has?** | Lung cancer |
| **Why?** | Cachectic appearance is consistent with malignancy, and patient is a smoker, which is the number one risk factor for lung cancer. |
| **What laboratory tests can be performed?** | CBC with platelet count and cell differential, renal and liver function tests, PT/PTT, sputum for culture, cytology |
| **Which diagnostic procedures should be performed first?** | CXR, possibly with a CT scan |
| **What other diagnostic tests may be helpful?** | Bronchoscopy |
| **How is mild hemoptysis treated?** | Control of cough. Reverse coagulopathy if present. Treat underlying disease. |
| **Which invasive procedures can be performed to treat hemoptysis?** | Bronchoscopy with topical epinephrine, balloon tamponade, cautery; bronchial arteriographic embolization; surgical resection |

## CASE 11

*A 62-year-old female presents to your clinic complaining of chest discomfort and shortness of breath. On physical examination, you find decreased tactile fremitus, dullness to percussion, and decreased breath sounds at the right lung base. You obtain an EKG, CXR, and basic labs. Results are unremarkable except for dullness of the right costophrenic angle.*

| | |
|---|---|
| **What are these findings consistent with?** | Pleural effusion |
| **How much fluid must accumulate before it can be noticed?** | At least 10 to 20 mL of fluid in the pleural space |
| **What imaging test will you order next?** | Lateral and decubitus x-ray to determine if it is free flowing |
| **What serum biochemistries should be ordered?** | Total protein, lactate dehydrogenase (LDH), glucose, triglycerides, and amylase |
| **What diagnostic procedure should be done?** | Diagnostic thoracocentesis to obtain pleural fluid for analysis |
| **Why?** | Results will narrow the differential of potential causes to transudates and exudates. |
| **What tests should be performed on aspirated pleural fluid?** | pH, LDH, protein, glucose, triglycerides, amylase, Gram stain, culture. AFB stain and mycobacterium culture if TB suspected. Cytology if malignancy suspected. |
| **How are transudative and exudative effusions differentiated?** | A pleural effusion is exudative if one of the following is present: pleural/serum protein >0.5, pleural/serum LDH >0.6, pleural LDH >2/3 upper limits of normal serum LDH. |

| | |
|---|---|
| **What are the causes of transudate?** | Congestive cardiac failure from any cause, hepatic cirrhosis, nephrotic syndrome, hypoalbuminemia, overhydration |
| **What are the causes of exudative pleural effusion?** | Infection, malignancy, pancreatitis, collagen vascular diseases, chylothorax, trauma, pulmonary embolism, drugs, chemical and irradiation injury |
| **What other lab tests should be performed if exudative effusion?** | White blood count, blood culture, erythrocyte sedimentation rate (ESR), serum antinuclear antibody level, PPD skin test |
| **What is the treatment for pleural effusions?** | Treat underlying cause, consider chest tube if effusion continues to expand or fluid is infected. |

## CASE 12

*A 65-year-old male with history of hypertension and aortic stenosis presents to your clinic after complaints of becoming short of breath while breathing fast after climbing a flight of stairs at a college football game. On exam you note basilar rales and faint wheezing without use of accessory respiratory muscles.*

| | |
|---|---|
| **What do the symptoms and signs suggest?** | Pulmonary edema |
| **What is his risk factor for pulmonary edema?** | Aortic stenosis |
| **What else can cause it?** | Left ventricular failure, MI, other valvular heart disease, arrhythmias, hypertensive crisis, volume overload, and ARDS |
| **What should be included in the workup?** | Chem 8, cardiac enzymes (rule out MI), CXR, ABG, EKG, and echocardiogram |

| | |
|---|---|
| **How is it diagnosed?** | CXR revealing diffuse bilateral interstitial and perihilar vascular engorgement, Kerley B lines (interlobar fluid and fibrosis), and possible pleural effusions |
| **What is the treatment?** | Correct underlying cause, diuretics (furosemide) and oxygen |

## CASE 13

*A 30-year-old African American female returns to your clinic for follow-up of fatigue, malaise, mild dyspnea, and a dry cough that gradually developed over the last few months. Her symptoms have not significantly improved and her physical exam is still significant for tender red nodules on the tibia. The CXR from last week reveals bilateral hilar adenopathy.*

| | |
|---|---|
| **What are you concerned about?** | Sarcoidosis |
| **What were the clues?** | African American (increased prevalence), tender red nodules on shin (consistent with erythema nodosum), and bilateral hilar adenopathy |
| **What other systemic clues could be presented to you?** | |
| **Eye and nervous system** | Uveitis, optic nerve dysfunction, Bell's (7th nerve) palsy |
| **Cardiac** | Cardiomyopathy, ventricular arrhythmias (including sudden death) |
| **What other organs can be involved?** | Joints (Migratory arthralgias and arthritis) |
| **What labs should be ordered?** | CMP, CBC, ACE level, ESR |

| | |
|---|---|
| **What lab abnormalities may be present?** | Mild lymphocytopenia, increased ACE and ESR, increased total protein (due to hypergammaglobulinemia) |
| **What PFT findings support the diagnosis?** | A restrictive pattern (decreased FEV1, FVC, TLC, and DLCO) is the most frequent. Can also show an obstructive pattern with a decreased FEV1/FVC ratio. |
| **How is the diagnosis made?** | Biopsy confirmation of noncaseating granulomas in affected organs (usually lung or skin). Other infectious or malignant causes must be ruled out. |
| **What's the treatment?** | Supportive at first because most cases spontaneously improve |
| **What if symptoms persist for 2–3 months?** | Prednisone taper |

## CASE 14

*A 47-year-old male with history of chronic bronchitis secondary to 20 pack years smoking and ESRD secondary to HTN and diabetes presents to your clinic after a 3.5-cm solitary lung nodule was found during routine tests for his kidney transplant evaluation.*

| | |
|---|---|
| **What is the basic differential for causes of solitary pulmonary nodule?** | Lung cancer (primary or metastatic), infectious and inflammatory |
| **What cause do you suspect in this patient?** | Primary lung cancer |
| **What clinical factors presented suggest a malignant solitary pulmonary nodule?** | Older age, smoking history, size over 3 cm |

| | |
|---|---|
| **What radiographic features suggest** | |
| **Benign etiology?** | Diffuse, central, laminated, or "popcorn" calcifications and stability of the size of the lesion over a period of at least 2 years |
| **Malignant?** | Irregular contour |
| **What is the first step in the evaluation?** | Review old chest x-rays to determine if this is a new lesion or old and stable process. |
| **What diagnostic procedures are available?** | CT-guided needle biopsy, fiberoptic bronchoscopy (washings and brushings for cytology and transbronchial biopsy) |
| **What is the treatment?** | |
| **Benign** | Follow with serial CXR to document stable lesion (not growing) |
| **Malignant** | Oncology and surgical consults to assess surgical, chemotherapeutic, and radiation-based therapies |

## CASE 15

*A 38-year-old postpartum female with history of obesity, asthma, smoking, hypertension, hyperlipidemia, and degenerative joint disease develops rapid onset of shortness of breath following a cross-country airline flight to visit her aging parents with her new baby. While pulling bags down from the overhead compartment she became breathless with rapid heart rate and breathing rate.*

| | |
|---|---|
| **What differential are you considering?** | MI, pneumothorax, pulmonary embolus, CHF, anxiety disorder with hyperventilation, asthma |
| **Which is most likely and why?** | Pulmonary embolus (PE) due to the acute symptoms onset and multiple risk factors present |

**What causes a PE?**

Blockage of a branch of the pulmonary artery by an embolus, often from a large vein, causing increased pulmonary artery pressure and right ventricular stain

**What symptoms and signs are suggestive of PE?**

In descending order of frequency: dyspnea, tachypnea, tachycardia, chest pain, cough, syncope, hemoptysis

**What risk factors for PE does she have?**

Postpartum and probable oral contraceptive use (most postpartum women are put on birth control by their ob-gyns), immobilized (plane ride), obesity, smoker

**What additional risk factors exist?**

Increased age, pregnancy, recent surgery, trauma, indwelling central venous catheter, cancer, coagulopathies

**What are the most common coagulopathies known to predispose to deep venous thrombosis?**

Activated protein C resistance (factor V Leiden), protein C deficiency, protein S deficiency, antithrombin III deficiency, plasminogen deficiency

**Where do pulmonary emboli commonly come from?**

Pelvic veins or deep veins of the legs

**What's the first step in managing this patient?**

Stabilize patient's vital signs by following basic ABCs (airway, breathing, and circulation) of cardiopulmonary resuscitation

**What initial tests should you order?**

Basic labs (chem 8, CBC, PT/PTT/INR), EKG, cardiac enzymes (Ck-MB and troponin), and ABG

**What one lab test can be ordered to help exclude PE from the differential diagnosis (high negative predictive value)?**

Negative plasma D-dimer by ELIZA (it is positive in roughly 90% of patients with PE)

**Would this be helpful in this patient?**

Probably not; she recently delivered a baby and likely has endogenous fibrinolysis occurring from that.

**So, when is the D-dimer test most helpful?**

In ruling out PE when your pre-test probability is low

**What may be found on ABG in PE?**

Increased alveolar-arterial oxygen gradient (measures difference in oxygen concentration between alveoli and arterial blood) and hypoxia (low $PaO_2$)

**What findings on the EKG suggest PE?**

New EKG changes of right ventricular strain with large S waves in leads I and aVL, QS waves in leads III and aVF, T wave inversions in leads III and aVF or $V_1$ through $V_4$

**What findings on CXR may be found days later suggesting prior PE?**

A peripheral wedge-shaped density (Hampton's hump) secondary to pulmonary infarction from a pulmonary embolus

**What ultrasound test can support the diagnosis of PE?**

Lower extremity Doppler US revealing a lower extremity deep venous thrombosis (LE DVT)

**What radiographic tests are commonly used to diagnose PE?**

V/Q scan (ventilation/perfusion scan) and spiral CT

**What does the V/Q scan do?**

Shows areas that are ventilated but not perfused

**What is the gold standard diagnostic test?**

Pulmonary angiography

**What's the treatment for PE?**

Supportive care and anticoagulation (IV heparin or LMWH followed by coumadin to keep INR between 2 and 3 for at least 3 months)

**What additional treatment may be required in massive PE?**

Thrombolysis or pulmonary embolectomy

## CASE 16

*A 17-year-old tall, thin male presents to the ER from school with splinting to his right side complaining of acute onset of dyspnea following smoking a cigarette after lunch. He says his right chest is killing him and wants some pain medication.*

| | |
|---|---|
| **What's your differential diagnosis?** | Pneumothorax, pleurisy, pulmonary embolism, MI, pericarditis, asthma, pneumonia |
| **Which is most likely?** | Pneumothorax based on his presentation and risk factors |
| **What is a pneumothorax?** | Accumulation of air in the pleural space with secondary lung collapse |
| **What is characteristic of pneumothorax?** | |
| Symptoms | Acute onset of dyspnea and chest pain (acute, localized to one side, usually pleuritic) |
| Signs | Tachycardia, tachypnea |
| **What physical exam findings would support your diagnosis?** | Absent tactile fremitus, hyperresonance, and decreased breath sounds on affected side (his right side) |
| **What are his risk factors for primary spontaneous pneumothorax?** | Male sex, tobacco use, tall and thin body habitus |
| **What are some secondary causes of pneumothorax (not suspected in this patient)?** | COPD, cystic fibrosis, HIV/AIDS, trauma, invasive procedures (central line placement, thoracentesis), mechanical ventilation |
| **What tests should you order?** | CXR and ABG |

**What results do you suspect on**

**ABG?**  Hypoxemia and hypocapnia (secondary to hyperventilation)

**CXR?**  A pleural line with absence of vessel markings peripheral to this line on the affected side (right)

**What test would you order if basic CXR was negative and you still suspected acute pneumothorax?**  CT of chest

**What is the usual treatment of pneumothorax?**  Aspiration of air using small IV catheter in second intercostal space in the mid-clavicular line connected to a large syringe; 100% oxygen. Follow with serial CXR to document resolution.

**When can a pneumothorax be observed?**  Asymptomatic patients with small pneumothorax (<15%) with evidence that the leak has sealed

**When is pleurodesis indicated?**  Recurrent primary spontaneous pneumothorax. Consider use in patients with COPD and HIV.

**When is surgery indicated?**  Persistent air leak, incomplete re-expansion of lung

**What complication would you suspect if the patient developed labored breathing, diaphoresis, cyanosis, distended neck veins, tracheal deviations, subcutaneous emphysema?**  Tension pneumothorax

**What's the physics behind a tension pneumothorax?**  Pleural pressure exceeds atmospheric pressure throughout expiration leading to compression of the mediastinum (heart and great vessels)

| | |
|---|---|
| **When is a tension pneumothorax most likely to occur?** | After trauma or during mechanical ventilation |
| **Why is a tension pneumothorax feared?** | Because it is associated with severe respiratory distress and hypotension |
| **What is the treatment?** | Prompt aspiration of air with a large bore needle |

## CASE 17

*A 30-year-old male presents to the ER after falling off his horse onto a tree stump. He becomes acutely short of breath and is splinting to his right side in excruciating pain. During inspiration, there is paradoxical inward movement of the flail segment, with outward movement of the segment during expiration.*

| | |
|---|---|
| **What diagnosis is associated with this paradoxical chest wall motion?** | Flail chest |
| **What risk factor is associated with it?** | Blunt trauma to the chest (like falling off a horse onto a tree stump) |
| **Why does the paradoxical motion occur?** | A segmental fracture (fractures in 2 or more locations on the same rib) of 3 or more adjacent ribs resulting in an unstable portion of the chest wall. Most often occurs anteriorly or laterally. |
| **Other than paradoxical motion, what other physical exam findings do you expect?** | Bony crepitus and tenderness |
| **What basic imaging test should you order to support your diagnosis?** | CXR |

**What is the appearance of the chest radiograph in a patient with flail chest?**

The fractured rib segments should be apparent, and there may be associated hemothorax or pneumothorax. Pulmonary contusion may be evident 6 hours after injury and appears as opacification of areas of the lung.

**How is it diagnosed?**

Physical exam

**What is the initial treatment of flail chest?**

Supplemental oxygen and analgesia

**What if severe hypoxemia or respiratory distress occurs?**

Mechanical ventilation

**Is surgical fixation of the ribs required?**

Rarely. Supportive treatment in the form of analgesia, supplemental oxygen, and mechanical ventilation as necessary are the mainstays of therapy.

**While hospitalized, he develops unilateral decreased breath sounds and dullness to chest percussion. What complication of flail chest do you suspect?**

Hemothorax

**What is a hemothorax?**

An accumulation of blood in one or both hemithoraces

**What is the cause of hemothorax?**

It is most often the result of penetrating chest trauma that disrupts systemic or hilar vessels, but may also occur as a result of blunt trauma.

**What lab tests should you order?**

CBC, PT, PTT, and INR

**What imaging test would help support the diagnosis?**

CXR

**In what position should the patient be for the CXR?**

Upright or decubitus

**Why?**

While an upright or decubitus chest radiograph may detect as little as 200 to 300 mL of fluid collection, as much as 1 L of fluid in the chest may be missed on a supine film.

**What is the treatment for a hemothorax?**

A tube thoracostomy (chest tube)

## CASE 18

*A 64-year-old male with history of hypertension, DJD, benign prostatic hypertrophy (BPH), and aortic stenosis s/p valve replacement presents to the ER after falling off his bike. He has been exercising for months, but lately has lost more weight than usual (30 pounds in 6 weeks) and has been easily fatigued within a mile of his ride. Other than some unsteadiness on his feet, productive cough which is infrequently bloody, and new thigh pain, he feels okay. CXR reveals hazy density in the hilum.*

**What's your differential diagnosis?**

Lung cancer, metastatic cancer, hamartoma, and granuloma (tuberculosis or fungal)

**What social history question is important to ask?**

Smoking history

**Why?**

Elderly male presenting with weight loss, hemoptysis, fatigue, and new neurologic complaints and bone pain is concerning for metastatic lung cancer, and smoking causes greater than 90% of all lung cancers.

**What other general symptoms of cancer should you ask about?**

Fever and weakness

**What additional respiratory signs and symptoms should you ask about?**

Dyspnea, chest pain, wheezing, stridor, hoarseness, and pleural effusion

**What metastatic symptom does he present with?**

Neurologic abnormalities (he is unsteady on his feet) and bone pain

**What basic lab tests should you order and why?**

CBC (look for anemia suggesting bone metastasis), Liver Function Test (LFT), PT, PTT, and platelet count (abnormalities suggest liver metastasis and need normal values if planning a biopsy in future)

**What additional radiographic tests should you order and why?**

CT scan of the chest (helps to define lung density and with cancer staging), CT of head (assess for metastatic lesions due to neurologic symptoms), and bone scan (due to new thigh pain suspicious for bony mets)

**CT of chest defines central lung mass and CT of head and bone scan have findings consistent with metastatic disease. What types of lung cancer present centrally on CXR and CT?**

Squamous cell carcinoma and small cell (oat cell) carcinoma

**Of the two, which is more likely in this patient?**

Small cell due to rapidly growing and virulent presentation

**Which lung tumors are peripherally located on the CXR?**

Adenocarcinoma and large cell carcinoma

**How will you make your diagnosis?**

Lung biopsy

**What biopsy procedures will the surgeons and interventional radiologists commonly use to obtain the lung tissue?**

Transbronchial biopsy, fine needle aspiration biopsy, thoracentesis, and thoracotomy

**Biopsy tissue confirms small cell cancer of the lung. What's the treatment?**

Chemotherapy, radiotherapy, immunotherapy, and pain relief when applicable

**When is surgery indicated?**　　In non-small cell lung cancer when chance of curative resection exists

**What paraneoplastic syn-drome may develop from this patient's small cell carcinoma?**　　Syndromes characterized by ACTH-like or antidiuretic hormone-like activity

# 3     Gastroenterology

## UPPER GI BLEEDING

### CASE I

*A 68-year-old male with history of gout, rheumatoid arthritis, coronary artery disease (CAD) s/p coronary artery bypass graft (CABG) 2 years ago, and abdominal aortic aneurysm (AAA) repair 4 years ago presents to your office complaining of progressive darkening of stool over last 3 weeks, one episode of vomiting with trace amount of bright red blood this morning, and mild shortness of breath (sob) with exertion.*

| | |
|---|---|
| **What's a reasonable differential diagnosis?** | Peptic ulcer disease (PUD), arteriovenous malformations (AVMs), aortoenteric fistula |
| **Which is most important to rule out in this patient?** | Aortoenteric fistula |
| **Why?** | Often the mild "sentinel," nonexsanguinating initial bleed, with blood per rectum (melena or hematochezia and hematemesis or with chronic intermittent bleeding) followed by a massive life-threatening hemorrhage |
| **What causes it?** | A fistula that forms after 2% of abdominal aortic grafts and is located usually between the upper portion of the aortic graft and the distal duodenum |
| **What key risk factor did this patient have?** | History of abdominal aortic aneurysm repair (4 years ago on average) |
| **What basic tests should be ordered first?** | CBC, PT and INR, EKG, CXR, hemoccult of stool, nasogastric (NG) lavage |

| | |
|---|---|
| **Hg 8, MCV 88, heme + stool, negative NG lavage, CXR, EKG, and PT and INR. What test should be ordered next to rule out aortoenteric fistula?** | Upper endoscopy |
| **What if endoscopy is not available?** | Angiography or abdominal CT scanning |
| **Upper endoscopy confirms the diagnosis of aortoenteric fistula. What is the treatment strategy?** | STAT surgical consult, transfuse with PRBC, serial Hg/hct, IV fluids, and antibiotics |
| **How can you explain the negative NG lavage?** | A clot formed within the fistula. |

## CASE 2

*A 73-year-old male with history of HTN, DJD, macular degeneration, and aortic stenosis (AS) presents to your clinic complaining of dark black sticky stools on and off for the last 2 months.*

| | |
|---|---|
| **What's a reasonable differential diagnosis?** | Aortoenteric fistula, angiodysplasia, PUD, gastric cancer |
| **Does the patient's history of AS help narrow your differential diagnosis?** | Yes, AS is associated with AVM. |
| **Name additional risk factors for AVMs.** | Age, chronic renal failure, hereditary hemorrhagic telangiectasia, von Willebrand disease, and scleroderma |
| **What causes AVMs?** | Abnormal arteriovenous communication that is hypothesized to arise from chronic intestinal muscular contractions obstructing venous mucosal drainage |
| **What are some other less common ways patients with AVMs present?** | Recurrent self-limited hematochezia, or hematemesis that is not hemodynamically significant |

| | |
|---|---|
| **Where do they most commonly occur?** | Colon (cecum and ascending colon) |
| **What other locations may be found in patients with chronic liver failure?** | Stomach and duodenum |
| **How is the diagnosis made?** | Endoscopically |
| **How is it treated?** | Iron supplementation with monitoring hemoglobin for response |
| **How is it treated if actively bleeding?** | Endoscopic coagulation |
| **What additional medical therapy may decrease recurrent bleeds?** | Combined estrogen and progesterone therapy |

## CASE 3

*A 51-year-old previously healthy male presents to your clinic with 30-pound weight loss over last 4 months, progressive difficulty swallowing food, and trace amounts of blood in vomited food over the last few days*

| | |
|---|---|
| **What diagnosis do you suspect?** | Esophageal cancer |
| **Why?** | Dysphagia, weight loss, vomiting, and hematemesis are characteristic of esophageal cancer. |
| **What other symptoms may a patient present with?** | Odynophagia, anorexia, cough, hoarseness, bone pain |
| **What is the most important question to ask the patient?** | "Do you drink alcohol and or use tobacco products?" |
| **Name the two most common types of esophageal cancer.** | Squamous cell carcinoma and adenocarcinoma |

| | |
|---|---|
| **Which is associated with ethyl alcohol (EtOH) and tobacco smoking?** | Squamous |
| **What is associated with adenocarcinoma of the esophagus?** | Barrett's esophagus from long-standing reflux disease |
| **What is the best diagnostic test?** | Endoscopy with biopsy |
| **What other test may be considered if endoscopy is unavailable?** | Barium esophagram |
| **Why is endoscopy preferred?** | Can obtain tissue for diagnosis |
| **What additional tests are performed for staging of the cancer?** | Staging requires CT of chest and abdomen, supplemented by endoscopic ultrasound and bone scan. |

## CASE 4

*A 62-year-old female with history of hypertension (HTN), diabetes mellitus (DM), degenerative joint disease (DJD), asthma, gastroesophageal reflux disease (GERD), and depression comes to the ER complaining of more frequent albuterol use for her asthma, hoarseness, and pain with swallowing.*

| | |
|---|---|
| **What's your differential diagnosis?** | Asthma exacerbation, GERD, esophagitis |
| **Is there a way that all three could be present?** | Yes |
| **What additional history would be helpful?** | Establishing a time-line of worsening reflux disease (heartburn; but can be asymptomatic), followed by more asthma attacks |
| **In addition to heartburn, what other symptoms of reflux esophagitis may be present?** | Regurgitation and water brash, which are aggravated on bending and lying down. Bleeding and dysphagia are seen owing to severe disease or complications. |

| | |
|---|---|
| **Why does GERD occur?** | Imbalance between the aggressive forces within the refluxate (acidic stomach contents) and the esophageal defenses constituted by the antireflux barriers, the luminal clearance mechanisms, and tissue resistance |
| **What are the most common causes of esophagitis (other than GERD) and esophageal ulcers?** | Radiation (history of thyroid cancer), pill-induced, chemical injury (lye), and infections (often in immunocompromised hosts) |
| **What's a reasonable diagnostic strategy?** | Medical therapy first, followed by upper endoscopy or ambulatory 24-hour intraesophageal pH monitoring if therapeutic trial unsuccessful |
| **What is the medical management of GERD?** | Lifestyle modification followed by treatment with proton pump inhibitors for 8–12 weeks |

## CASE 5

*A 44-year-old male with known hepatitis C and EtOH cirrhosis confirmed by recent liver biopsy, ascites, HTN, DJD, stomach ulcers, and pancreatitis comes by ambulance to your ER with 4 episodes of large quantity of bright red emesis over the last 3 hours, and 1 recent episode of dark stool.*

| | |
|---|---|
| **What's your differential diagnosis?** | Esophageal varices, Mallory-Weiss tears, PUD |
| **Which is most likely?** | Esophageal varices |
| **Why?** | Patient has known cirrhosis of liver |
| **What causes varices to develop?** | When portal hypertension develops in cirrhotics, extrahepatic collateral venous channels between portal and systemic circulation dilate and form varices, most often in the lower esophagus. |
| **What's the first management step for this patient?** | STAT labs (CBC, coags, Chem 8, LFTs), stabilize patient with IVF and PRBC |

| | |
|---|---|
| **What's the next step?** | Upper endoscopy for diagnosis and treatment |
| **What additional therapy is used to reduce portal pressures?** | Octreotide |
| **What if this management fails?** | Order surgical consult for Transjugular Intrahepatic Portosystemic Shunt (TIPPS) evaluation |
| **After acute bleed is stabilized and patient is hemodynamically stable, what prophylactic medication is useful?** | β-blockers (decrease portal pressure) |

## CASE 6

*A 47-year-old African American female with history of severe peptic ulcer disease requiring Billroth II 18 years ago presents to the ER with complaints of persistent and progressive abdominal pain, weight loss, and early satiety over the last 7 weeks.*

| | |
|---|---|
| **What's a reasonable differential diagnosis?** | Cancer (gastric, esophageal), PUD |
| **Which is most likely?** | Gastric cancer |
| **Name some common presenting signs and symptoms of gastric cancer** | Weight loss, abdominal pain (often constant), dyspepsis, early satiety, anorexia, hematemesis, or melena |
| **What risk factors does she have for gastric cancer?** | African American and Billroth II |
| **What additional risk factors are there for gastric cancer?** | Family history, hereditary (Asian Americans, Hispanics), gastric polyps, and possibly chronic *Helicobacter pylori* gastritis |
| **What lab tests would support your suspicion of gastric cancer?** | Iron-deficient anemia (chronic blood loss), positive guaiac test (50%), and positive carcinoembryonic antigen (CEA) |

| | |
|---|---|
| **Which abnormal lab result would raise suspicion of metastasis?** | Abnormal liver chemistry tests |
| **What basic imaging test would help support the diagnosis?** | Upper GI series |
| **What's the best test to make the diagnosis?** | Upper endoscopy with biopsy |
| **An upper endoscopy is performed; findings and biopsy results are consistent with gastric cancer. What histologic type of gastric cancer is most likely?** | Adenocarcinoma (90–95%); others include leiomyosarcoma (common cause of massive UGI bleed) and lymphoma |
| **What additional imaging should be ordered now?** | Abdominal and chest CT for staging |
| **What is the therapy?** | Surgical resection for localized disease; chemotherapy and radiation may also be used as adjunctive and palliative therapy. |

## CASE 7

*A 44-year-old female with history of HTN, diabetes, COPD, and chronic back pain controlled with ibuprofen was admitted to the hospital 7 days ago after a motor vehicle collision, with significant blood loss that required a splenectomy. She continues to be on the ventilator owing to difficulty in weaning as a result of underlying COPD. You are called to evaluate 2 episodes of coffee ground emesis.*

| | |
|---|---|
| **What's a reasonable differential diagnosis?** | Esophageal ulcers and esophagitis, hemorrhagic gastritis, and peptic ulcer disease |
| **Which do you suspect?** | Hemorrhagic gastritis (HG) or PUD |
| **What is HG?** | An inflammatory hemorrhagic mucosal erosion in the stomach often caused by noxious chemical agents or physiologic stress eroding viable tissue |

**What is PUD?**

A lesion in the gastric or duodenal mucosa that arises when normal mucosal defenses are impaired or are overwhelmed by aggressive luminal factors such as acid or pepsin

**What risk factors does this patient have for HG and PUD?**

NSAID use, physiologic stress of underlying illness

**Name other risk factors for both HG and PUD.**

Aspirin, NSAIDs, alcohol, physiologic stress, trauma (endoscopy, nasogastric tubes)

**How do they commonly present?**
    **HG**

Often asymptomatic, but may present with dyspepsia; mild cases present with epigastric pain, anorexia, nausea and vomiting; if severe (rare), hematemesis or coffee ground emesis, bloody aspirate in nasogastric tube, or melena

    **PUD**

Gnawing/burning epigastric pain (duodenal ulcers are relieved by food while gastric often are not), hematemesis, melena, or coffee ground emesis

**What's the first thing to do with this patient?**

Determine how severe the bleeding is

**What are some physical exam signs in cases of significant blood loss?**

Pale, diaphoretic, tachycardia, hypotension and dizziness, melena, hematemesis, and orthostatic symptoms

**What lab test is helpful?**

Hematocrit (anemia), stool for occult blood or guaiac test

**What bedside test helps determine if the patient is still actively bleeding?**

NG lavage and aspirate looking for fresh blood (may be false negative if bleed is post-pyloric)

**What is the most sensitive diagnostic test?**

Upper endoscopy

| | |
|---|---|
| **What else should be done during endoscopy?** | Antral biopsy for *H. pylori* |
| **What distinguishes the erosions seen in gastritis from those in PUD and HG?** | Erosions in gastritis are less than 5 mm in diameter and do not extend through the muscularis mucosa. |
| **What is the initial therapy in massive GI bleeds?** | Stabilize the patient with fluid resuscitation and packed red blood cells as needed; if bleeding continues consider intravenous vasopressin or endoscopic control. Surgical intervention may be required. |
| **What additional treatment is required?** | Antisecretory therapy ($H_2$ receptor antagonists or a proton pump inhibitor); treatment for *H. pylori* if present, may add sucralfate to therapy regimen especially when NSAID or stress induced; discontinue alcohol and chronic NSAID use |

## CASE 8

*A 22-year-old alcoholic is transferred by ambulance to the ER after being found on the grounds of a fraternity house with dried blood with food particles on his mouth and shirt. Friends told EMS personnel that he was not feeling well earlier and said he felt nauseous and he was going to get sick.*

| | |
|---|---|
| **What is the most likely cause of the bleeding?** | Mallory-Weiss tear |
| **Why?** | Classically, patients present after repeated, violent retching, vomiting, or coughing followed by hematemesis. |
| **What is the cause?** | Sudden rise of intra-abdominal pressure that produces a linear, nonpenetrating mucosal laceration at the gastro-esophageal junction resulting in bleeding |
| **How is the diagnosis made?** | Endoscopy is the preferred modality for diagnosis. |

| | |
|---|---|
| **What are the treatment options?** | Most stop bleeding spontaneously. If bleeding persists, endoscopic hemostasis can be attempted by injecting epinephrine or by cauterization. |

## LOWER GI BLEEDING

### CASE 9

*A 55-year-old female with history of ulcerative colitis, hepatitis C secondary to IVDA in her teens, and adenomatous colon polyps removed on a flexible sigmoidoscope 12 years ago presents with unexplained weight loss, lower left quadrant abdominal pressure, fatigue and change in bowel habits, and trace amounts of blood on tissue paper.*

| | |
|---|---|
| **What diagnosis is most likely?** | Colorectal cancer (CRC) |
| **Why?** | Recent change in bowel habits, abdominal pain, rectal bleeding, and weight loss are concerning for CRC. |
| **What risk factor does she have for CRC?** | Adenomatous polyps and ulcerative colitis |
| **What additional risk factors are there?** | Family history of colon cancer, other adenocarcinomas (breast, ovarian, etc.) |
| **What does CRC most commonly arise from?** | Adenomatous polyps (villous polyps are more often malignant than tubular polyps) |
| **What physical exam clues may be found in CRC patients?** | Pale skin and conjunctivae (anemia), palpable abdominal or rectal mass, blood on rectal exam, or heme-positive stool |
| **What lab test result would support the diagnosis?** | Iron-deficient anemia (microcytic anemia with low iron, ferritin, and high total iron binding capacity) |
| **How is the diagnosis made?** | Colonoscopy with biopsy |

| | |
|---|---|
| **After the diagnosis is made, what additional radiographic studies are often performed?** | CXR, bone scan (if patient complains of bone pain), and abdominal CT scan |
| **What is the treatment?** | Surgically resect cancer (if rectal cancer, consider preoperative radiation therapy), adjuvant therapy with 5-FU, and leucovorin may be used in locally advanced and metastatic cases. |

## CASE 10

*A 62-year-old female with history of chronic constipation, type 2 diabetes, and psoriasis presents to the ER with 3 episodes of 300 cc of painless bright red bleeding per rectum since this morning.*

| | |
|---|---|
| **What's your differential diagnosis?** | Hemorroids, diverticulosis, and anal fissure |
| **Which is most likely?** | Diverticulosis |
| **Why?** | Painless rectal bleeding (large volume bright red to maroon blood) with chronic constipation or crampy postprandial pain in the left lower quadrant, dark red stool common, possibly light-headedness (if hemodynamically unstable) are characteristic of diverticulosis. |
| **Why are hemorrhoids and anal fissure less likely?** | Rarely do these conditions present with a large quantity of blood as seen in this patient. |
| **What causes diverticulosis?** | Pouch-like herniations through the muscular layer of the colon (usually sigmoid) around a diverticular arteriole leading to bright red bleeding per rectum |
| **What risk factors did this patient have for diverticulosis?** | Age 60 or older and chronic constipation |
| **What basic physical exam studies should be performed?** | Check vital signs for orthostatics (assess degree of blood loss) and stool guaiac test |

| | |
|---|---|
| **What laboratory tests should be ordered?** | CBC, type and cross |
| **What diagnostic studies should be ordered?** | Proctosigmoidoscope or colonoscopy to identify bleeding as left sided and confirm that no other lesions are present |
| **Can proctosigmoidoscope or colonoscopy reveal the source of the bleeding?** | Usually not, because the bleeding tends to obscure the visual field |
| **What is the therapy in hemodynamically stable patients?** | Supportive (most bleeding spontaneously resolves) and high-fiber diet |
| **What is the therapy in hemodynamically unstable patients?** | Colonoscopy with angiographic control with intra-arterial vasopressin injection |
| **What if bleeding recurs despite above measures?** | Consider surgical resection |

## CASE 11

*A 35-year-old overweight sedentary previously healthy male presents to your office complaining of scant amounts of bright red blood on the tissue paper and a slight red tinge to toilet bowel water. He also says when he wipes the skin it's bumpy and itches afterwards.*

| | |
|---|---|
| **What differential diagnosis are you considering?** | Hemorrhoids and anal fissure |
| **Which is most likely?** | Hemorrhoids due to "bumpy" description and anal pruritis (not found with anal fissure) |
| **What causes hemorrhoids?** | Swelling and dilatation of a blood vessel at the anus most likely caused by increased vascular pressure |
| **What are the risk factors?** | Straining at stool, constipation, prolonged sitting, congestive heart failure, portal hypertension, pregnancy, obesity, and low-fiber diets |

| | |
|---|---|
| **What might the rectal examination reveal?** | Bluish tense lumps of skin that may be painful (external hemorrhoids are painful whereas internal ones are not) |
| **What diagnostic study is ordered?** | Rectal exam and proctosigmoidoscopy to reveal red blood and bleeding hemorrhoid |

**What is the treatment strategy in**

| | |
|---|---|
| **Asymptomatic patients?** | High-fiber diet, increase fluid intake, and physical activity |
| **Symptomatic patients?** | Sitz baths, topical itch and pain ointments, and oral analgesics if necessary |
| **Severe cases unresponsive to medical therapy?** | Banding, ligation, and cauterization |

## CASE 12

A 22-year-old female with 12 months history of intermittent crampy right lower quadrant abdominal pain, loose, nonbloody stools, and 10-pound weight loss presents to the ER with worsening pain unresponsive to over-the-counter pain medications.

| | |
|---|---|
| **What differential are you considering before examining the patient?** | Acute appendicitis, incarcerated hernia, inflammatory bowel disease, intestinal obstruction, ectopic pregnancy, ovarian cyst, torsion of ovarian cyst, salpingitis, tubo-ovarian abscess, kidney stone, and pyelonephritis |
| **On physical exam you find normal vital signs, but are impressed with bilateral red eyes, aphthous mouth ulcers, and right lower quadrant (RLQ) tenderness. Does this narrow your differential?** | Yes, the red eye (suggests possible iritis) and aphthous ulcers are extraintestinal manifestations of inflammatory bowel disease. |

**What other extraintestinal clues suggest inflammatory bowel disease?**

Uveitis, arthritis, or erythema nodosum

**What are the two inflammatory bowel diseases?**

Crohns and ulcerative colitis

**What symptoms may present in both?**

Abdominal pain, weight loss, fever, chills, nausea, and vomiting

**What are the characteristic symptoms of ulcerative colitis?**

Bloody diarrhea (classic) with tenesmus

**What is the classic symptom of Crohn disease?**

Nonbloody diarrhea

**Which is more likely here?**

Crohn disease

**Why?**

RLQ (suggest possible terminal ileum involvement characteristic of Crohn disease) and nonbloody diarrhea suggest Crohn disease.

**What basic labs should be ordered?**

UA (rule out renal causes), B-Hcg (rule out pregnancy), Chem 8, CBC

**What imaging test could be considered?**

CT scan with PO and IV contrast looking for bowel wall thickening suggestive of inflammation and underlying inflammatory bowel disease (IBD)

**What diagnostic study is ordered?**

Colonoscopy with biopsy and slit light exam (due to eye redness, rule out iritis)

**What is the characteristic distribution in Crohn disease?**

It can effect any region of the GI tract from the mouth to the anus with skip lesions with asymmetric ulceration, cobblestoning, and aphthous ulcers and does not usually effect the rectum. Affects the terminal ileum in 70% of cases.

**What is the characteristic distribution in ulcerative colitis?**

Usually starts in the rectum and spreads proximally in a symmetric and continuous fashion

| | |
|---|---|
| **Colonoscopy confirms terminal ileum involvement. What's your diagnosis?** | Crohn disease |
| **What medications are used to treat mild or moderately active disease and to maintain a remission in IBD?** | Sulfasalazine (decrease chronic inflammation) and mesalamine (use if intolerant to sulfasalazine) |
| **What drug can be added for acute exacerbations?** | Glucocorticoids (for acute exacerbations) in both oral and topical forms |
| **When is surgery warranted in ulcerative colitis?** | In life-threatening conditions (severe ongoing hemorrhage, toxic megacolon, or cancer) |
| **What additional medication can be used in moderately severe Crohn disease patients?** | TNF-α inhibitors, e.g., infliximab (Remicade) |
| **When might surgery be considered in Crohn disease?** | After medical therapy has failed in treating fistulas, obstruction, abscess, perforation, or severe ongoing hemorrhage |
| **What is the curative treatment for ulcerative colitis?** | Total proctocolectomy and ileostomy |

## CASE 13

*A 72-year-old male with history of HTN, DM, PVD, CAD s/p CABG 4 years ago presents with low-grade fever, abdominal pain, and bright red blood per rectum. Abdomen is nontender and bowel sounds hypoactive.*

| | |
|---|---|
| **What do you suspect?** | Ischemic bowel disease caused by blood supply to the small intestine or colon |
| **How do patients present with ischemic bowel disease?** | Low-grade fever, bloody diarrhea or hematochezia, and left lower quadrant tenderness |
| **What are his risk factors for ischemic bowel disease?** | Old age, atherosclerotic disease, peripheral vascular disease |

| | |
|---|---|
| **What additional risk factor is there?** | Hypercoagulable states |
| **What imaging study should you order?** | CT scan of the abdomen and pelvis looking for bowel wall edema and air (pneumatosis intestinalis) |
| **CT reveals pneumatosis intestinalis. What diagnostic study is ordered next?** | Flexible sigmoidoscope or colonoscopy |
| **What risk is associated with endoscopy?** | Perforation |
| **What is the therapy?** | Correct underlying causes of low flow states; no specific therapy is effective. |

## DIARRHEA

### CASE 14

*A 14-year-old girl previously healthy presents with acute onset of nausea, vomiting, abdominal cramping, and nonbloody diarrhea after coming home from a family picnic yesterday. She has had 8 nonbloody bowel movements in the last 24 hours.*

| | |
|---|---|
| **What type of infection is most likely?** | Acute noninflammatory diarrhea |
| **How does noninflammatory diarrhea present?** | Watery, nonbloody diarrhea with associated cramps, bloating, nausea, and/or vomiting; no fever or leukocytosis |
| **What causative organism do you suspect?** | *Staphylococcus aureus* |
| **Why?** | *S. aureus* is associated with food poisoning and prominent vomiting. |
| **What other organism is associated with prominent vomiting?** | Viruses (Norwalk and rotavirus) |

**What organism is associated with**

**Recent travel (especially Mexico)?** ETEC

**Sexually transmission?** *Giardia*

**Seafood ingestion?** *Vibrio cholerae*

**What lab tests at a minimum should you order?** CBC (rule out leukocytosis), Chem 8 (assess electrolytes and evidence of dehydration), stool for occult blood, fecal leukocytes (rule out infectious cause)

**How is the diagnosis made?** Negative examination of stool for fecal leukocytes and blood

**What is the treatment?** Oral rehydration and antidiarrheal agents (loperamide) for mild to moderate cases, supportive otherwise

## CASE 15

*A 10-year-old previously healthy boy returns from India with his mother and comes down with a low-grade fever and bloody diarrhea.*

**What type of diarrhea do you suspect?** Inflammatory diarrhea due to fever and bloody diarrhea

**Which organism do you suspect?** *Entamoeba histolytica*

**Why?** It's associated with recent travel (especially Asia, India, South and Central America).

**What other clues to the diagnosis should you look out for?**

**Dysentery-like illness days after food ingestion** *Shigella*

**Dairy product or eggs** *Salmonella*

**Food poisoning** *Campylobacter*

| | |
|---|---|
| **Recent antibiotic use** | *Clostridium difficile* |
| **Contaminated meat products and hemolytic-uremic syndrome** | EHEC 0157:H7 |
| **Immunocompromised and HIV-infected patients** | Cytomegalovirus |
| **What basic lab test will you order to make the diagnosis of infectious diarrhea?** | Fecal leukocytes (should be positive) |
| **What additional tests are required to diagnose Shigella, Salmonella, Campylobacter, and EHEC 0157:H7?** | Stool culture |
| ***Entamoeba histolytica?*** | Wet mount examination of stool for amebiasis |
| ***Clostridium difficile?*** | *C. difficile* toxin in the stool or demonstration of pseudomembranes on sigmoidoscopy |
| ***Giardia?*** | Stool parasite exam or duodenal aspirate exam if stool is negative |
| **What is the initial treatment strategy?** | Rehydration if necessary and empiric antibiotic treatment with ciprofloxacin, trimethoprim-sulfamethoxazole, or erythromycin while awaiting culture results |
| **What's the specific therapy for** | |
| ***C. difficile?*** | Metronidazole |
| ***Salmonella, Shigella,* and *Campylobacter?*** | Ciprofloxacin |
| ***Cytomegalovirus?*** | Ganciclovir |
| ***Entamoeba histolytica?*** | Metronidazole |

## HEPATIC INFLAMMATION

### CASE 16

*A 50-year-old previously healthy male decides to see a doctor for the first time since his service in the military due to his wife's urging. The physical exam is unremarkable except for hepatomegaly 2 cm below the costal margin. His liver chemistry tests are abnormal with an AST of 250 and ALT of 88.*

| | |
|---|---|
| **What's the first question you are going to ask the patient?** | "How much EtOH do you drink?" |
| **Why?** | ↑ AST (<500), ↑ AST/ALT (3:1) is associated with alcoholic liver disease. |
| **What other lab abnormalities may be present?** | ↑ MCV, ↑ WBC, and ↑ Bilirubin |
| **What course in the disease do you suspect the patient is in?** | Early (often asymptomatic with abnormal liver enzyme tests) |
| **What are some signs and symptoms of alcoholic cirrhosis?** | Weakness, fatigue, weight loss, jaundice, hepatomegaly, ascites, palmar erythema, spider angiomata, varices, and testicular atrophy |
| **How is the diagnosis made?** | History, presentation, and associated liver enzyme tests; liver biopsy may confirm it (shows fat, PMNs, and hyaline) |
| **What is the therapy?** | Discontinue all alcoholic beverages, vitamin and nutritional support |
| **When is transplant recommended?** | In end-stage cirrhotic liver disease with at least 6 months abstinence from alcohol |

### CASE 17

*A 37-year-old nonsmoking female is diagnosed with emphysematous lung disease after complaining of shortness of breath and wheezing to her primary care physician. The cause of the lung disease is unclear. On a follow-up visit, her symptoms have decreased on therapy. But now the lab reports that there is mild to moderate elevation of her liver chemistry tests suggestive of hepatitis.*

| | |
|---|---|
| **Which underlying disease do you suspect?** | α-1 antitrypsin deficiency because the patient is a young nonsmoker with emphysema of unknown cause presenting with abnormal liver chemistry tests |
| **What organs can α-1 antitrypsin deficiency affect?** | Lungs, liver, and pancreas |
| **Do all patients with liver disease have the associated pulmonary emphysema?** | No |
| **What is α-1 antitrypsin?** | A plasma protein produced in the liver that inhibits proteolytic enzymes like trypsin |
| **What lab tests support the diagnosis?** | Positive ZZ genotype test or low levels of α-1 antitrypsin (low levels alone are not diagnostic; may be heterozygous) |
| **How is the diagnosis confirmed?** | Liver biopsy |
| **What is the treatment?** | Supportive |
| **What treatment should be considered if end-stage liver disease develops?** | Liver transplant because it is curative by correcting the underlying metabolic defect |

## CASE 18

*A 58-year-old female with history of hypothyroidism, diabetes, and hypercholesteremia presents for follow-up office visit after noting 3× elevation of her alanine aminotransference (ALT) and aspartate transaminase (AST) 4 weeks ago. At that time, you discontinued the cholesterol-lowering medication and it had no effect. Viral hepatitis was also ruled out.*

| | |
|---|---|
| **What disease should be first on your differential diagnosis based on her history?** | Autoimmune hepatitis (AIH) |
| **Why?** | Female (more common) with other autoimmune disease presenting with elevated liver chemistries is suspicious for AIH. |

| | |
|---|---|
| **Name 4 associated lab findings that are helpful in making the diagnosis.** | Any or all of the following may be positive: anti-smooth muscle antibody, antinuclear antibody, hypergammaglobulinemia (IgG), and anti-liver-kidney-microsomal antibody. |
| **How is it diagnosed?** | Liver biopsy |
| **What is the treatment?** | Prednisone and azathioprine |

## CASE 19

A 28-year-old alcoholic with chronic pancreatitis presents for follow-up after starting Alcoholics Anonymous. She continues to drink, but has cut back to one six-pack per day. She complains of lower pack pain that started after lifting her child into his car seat 1 week ago. Her physical exam is unremarkable, but there is significant elevation of her ALT and AST to around 1000 U/L.

| | |
|---|---|
| **What are the common causes of ALT greater than 1000?** | Ischemia (recent shock), toxins, drugs, gallstones in biliary tree, viral and autoimmune hepatitis |
| **Which is most likely here?** | Drug induced |
| **What was the clue in the presentation?** | Recent back pain |
| **What's the most likely and most common offending drug to cause this?** | Acetaminophen |
| **Are excessive doses of acetaminophen required to cause acute liver failure in an alcoholic?** | No, therapeutic dosing can cause it. |
| **Name some other prescribed drugs that cause severe elevations of AST and ALT.** | Isoniazid, phenytoin, 6-mercaptopurine, valproic acid, nitrofurantoin, and ketoconazole |
| **What are patients at risk of?** | Acute liver failure |

**What are some symptoms of acetaminophen-induced acute liver failure?**

    **Early (0–24 hours)**    GI irritation (nausea, vomiting, and anorexia), lethargy, diaphoresis

    **Late (3–4 days) after ingestion**    Progressive hepatic encephalopathy (including confusion, lethargy, and coma) indicating fulminant hepatic failure

**What additional liver tests are critical to determine severity of underlying injury?**    Bilirubin and PT or INR

**What serum test should you order to determine treatment strategy?**    Acetaminophen level

**What is the treatment in general for drug hepatotoxicity?**    Discontinue medication; consider liver transplant if patient develops fulminant hepatic failure.

**What is the treatment for acetaminophen toxicity?**    Gastric decontamination using ipecac or gastric lavage, activated charcoal, cathartic, and N-acetylcysteine (antidote)

## CASE 20

*A 55-year-old white male with history of arthritis, diabetes, and dark complexion presents to your clinic after being declined life insurance due to abnormal AST and ALT of around 200 U/L. Physical exam is unremarkable except for mild hepatomegaly 1 cm below the right costal margin and tanned skin.*

**What underlying liver disease do you suspect?**    Hemochromatosis

**Why?**    Dark complexion (bronze color, tanned appearance), diabetes, and arthritis were clues in the presentation.

**What other clues may be presented to you if the patient is male?**    Hypogonadism

| | |
|---|---|
| **In practice (real life), how do most patients actually present?** | Asymptomatic |
| **What causes hemochromatosis?** | A common inherited autosomal recessive disorder of iron metabolism that results in excess iron deposits throughout the body |
| **What lab tests will you order to support your diagnosis?** | A fasting serum transferrin saturation (above 45% suggests the disease) |
| **How is the diagnosis confirmed?** | Increased iron weight on liver biopsy |
| **What's the therapy?** | Phlebotomy or deferoxamine (iron chelating agent) if unable to tolerate phlebotomy |

## CASE 21

*A previously healthy 17-year-old female returns from vacation with friends and develops progressive nausea and anorexia followed by yellow skin and eyes and dark urine. Her mother calls her friend's mom in the nearby town and learns that there has been an outbreak of this in the last week.*

| | |
|---|---|
| **What the most likely cause?** | Hepatitis A virus (HAV) |
| **How did she get it?** | Probably via fecal-oral route from contaminated food or water |
| **What are the risk factors for hepatitis A infection?** | Recent travel to endemic areas, children in day care, eating raw shellfish |
| **What lab tests should be performed?** | HAV IgM and IgG serum antibody tests, liver function tests (AST and ALT), alkaline phosphatase, and bilirubin |
| **How is the diagnosis of acute hepatitis A made?** | HAV IgM serum antibody test |
| **What lab test indicates previous exposure to HAV and immunity to recurring HAV infection?** | A positive HAV IgG serum antibody test |

| | |
|---|---|
| **What is the treatment?** | Supportive. HAV immune globulin should be given to all close personal contacts of patients with hepatitis A. |

## CASE 22

*A 44-year-old thin, healthy female married to a man with chronic hepatitis B presents for follow-up after yearly physical exam. You are concerned about mild elevations of her ALT and AST, around 220 U/L. She denies alcohol use, she is thin, denies prior IVDA, tattoos, blood transfusions, or family history of liver disease.*

| | |
|---|---|
| **What can cause these mild elevations?** | Medications, hepatitis B and C, hemochromatosis, fatty liver, autoimmune hepatitis, Wilson disease, and $\alpha$-1 antitrypsin disease |
| **What is the most likely cause?** | Hepatitis B |
| **How does it present?** | Often asymptomatic (80%), but a prodrome of nausea, anorexia, and malaise followed by jaundice, dark urine, and abdominal pain may occur. |
| **What causes it?** | Hepatitis B virus (HBV), a DNA virus |
| **How is it transmitted?** | Usually via contaminated blood or sexual contact (her husband has chronic hepatitis B) |
| **What are the risk factors for hepatitis B?** | Injection drug users and men who have sex with men, native Asians, health care workers, tattoos, and vertical transmission in pregnancy |
| **How is diagnosis of acute hepatitis B made?** | Positive hepatitis B surface antigen (HBsAg) and hepatitis B core antibody from the IgM class (IgM anti-HBcAb) |
| **What treatment is available for patients recently exposed to HBV?** | Hepatitis B immunoglobulin (HBIG) |

| | |
|---|---|
| **What is the medical treatment for acute hepatitis B?** | Supportive |
| **What is the medical treatment for chronic (at least 6 months) hepatitis B?** | α-interferon subcutaneous injections or oral lamivudine or adefovir |

## CASE 23

*A 49-year-old male lead singer for a well-known rock band is found to have elevated ALT and AST of around 180 U/L on routine lab tests. He admits to IVDA in the past and alcohol use, but quit drinking 10 years ago. He has made significant changes in his life and has been routinely exercising and eating well.*

| | |
|---|---|
| **What is the most likely cause of his abnormal liver chemistry tests?** | Hepatitis C |
| **Why?** | IVDA is a risk factor for hepatitis C infection, and he has mild elevation of his liver chemistry tests, which is characteristic of the disease. |
| **What other risk factors are there?** | Transfusion recipients (before 1992), health care workers, tattoos |
| **How is it usually transmitted?** | Via contaminated blood transfusions or needles |
| **How can it present?** | Majority are asymptomatic, but a prodrome of nausea, anorexia, and malaise followed by jaundice, dark urine, and abdominal pain may occur. |
| **What causes it?** | Hepatitis C virus (HCV), an RNA virus |
| **What lab tests should you order?** | Hepatitis C serum antibody test, PCR RNA for hepatitis C, liver function tests (AST and ALT), alkaline phosphatase, and bilirubin |
| **Which test indicates prior infection?** | Hepatitis C antibody |

| | |
|---|---|
| **What test indicates ongoing viral infection?** | PCR for hepatitis C RNA |
| **What is the treatment for chronic hepatitis C (greater than 6 months)?** | α-interferon with oral ribavirin for 6–12 months |

## CASE 24

*A 55-year-old male with history of CAD admitted to the hospital with a cardiac arrest secondary to acute MI is now stabilized in the ICU on pressor medications to sustain adequate blood pressure. On a routine blood draw, you note new elevations of his ALT and AST to 1200 U/L.*

| | |
|---|---|
| **What's the most likely cause?** | Ischemic hepatitis secondary to hypotension during cardiac arrest |
| **What are the risk factors for ischemic hepatitis?** | Low-flow states [shock (often unwitnessed and undocumented), congestive heart failure (CHF), MI, and arrhythmia] |
| **How is it diagnosed?** | History of low-flow state (transient hypotension) preceding rapid rise of transaminases into the thousands |
| **What is the therapy?** | Supportive, correct underlying low-flow state |

## CASE 25

*A 24-year-old previously healthy male comes to you because he is having difficulty walking. Physical exam is impressive for golden brown deposits in the cornea and a parkinsonian-like tremor.*

| | |
|---|---|
| **What's your most likely diagnosis?** | Wilson disease |
| **What were the clues in the presentation?** | Young adult with tremor and golden brown corneal deposits |
| **How can Wilson disease present?** | As liver disease in adolescents and neuropsychiatric disease in young adults |

| | |
|---|---|
| **What are the golden brown corneal deposits called in Wilson disease?** | Kaiser-Fleisher rings |
| **What other neurologic findings may be found on physical exam?** | Rigidity and chorea-type movements (common by age 40) |
| **What psychiatric findings may be found on physical exam?** | Depression and psychosis |
| **What causes Wilson disease?** | An autosomal recessive disorder of copper metabolism characterized by progressive copper accumulation in the liver which is then released and taken up by other organs (brain, cornea, kidney, etc.) |
| **Why does the copper accumulate in the liver?** | It is unable to excrete sufficient copper into the bile. |
| **What lab tests and physical exam finding support the diagnosis?** | Elevated 24-hour urinary copper levels, low serum ceruloplasmin, and Kaiser-Fleisher rings |
| **How is the diagnosis confirmed?** | Increased copper weight on liver biopsy |
| **What is the medical treatment?** | Lifelong copper-chelating agents (penicillamine) |

## CHOLESTATIC DISEASE

CASE 26

A 41-year-old alcoholic male presents to the ER again with complaints of abdominal pain that radiates to his back and stools that float in the toilet bowl after drinking large quantities of alcohol. The character of the pain is similar to prior episodes, but is more prolonged this time. He knows alcohol binging worsens his condition, but he just can't stop drinking.

| | |
|---|---|
| **What's the most likely cause of his abdominal pain?** | Acute or chronic pancreatitis secondary to alcohol |

**What other condition causes epigastric pain radiating to the back?**

Penetrating PUD

**Why is pancreatitis more likely?**

Patient describes steatorrhea (stools that float) which supports pancreatitis and exocrine insufficiency

**What other symptoms may patients with pancreatitis present with?**

Jaundice, diabetes, and weight loss

**What are common risk factors for pancreatitis?**

Chronic alcoholism and history of gallstone disease

**What's the basic underlying mechanism of disease?**

Inflammation of the pancreas from scarring or stricture of the distal common bile duct

**What labs are consistent with pancreatitis?**

Elevated amylase and lipase

**Can these be normal in pancreatitis?**

Yes

**When?**

Patchy focal disease or significant underlying fibrosis/scarring

**What tests can be done on the stool to diagnose pancreatic exocrine dysfunction?**

Quantitative fecal fat ($>7$ g of fat per day), qualitative fecal fat (Sudan test), and stool elastase 1

**What imaging studies are helpful in making the diagnosis?**

US (rule out gallstones or dilated biliary tree), CT scan (visualize pancreas), and ERCP (visualize pancreatic duct)

**What findings on US and CT are consistent with pancreatitis?**

Pancreatic calcifications, enlargement, ductal dilatation, and pseudocysts (fluid collection around the pancreas)

**What other important disease will CT and US help rule out as a cause of this patient's exacerbation?**

Pancreatic cancer

| | |
|---|---|
| **What additional diagnostic test can be ordered if CT and US are inconclusive?** | ERCP |
| **What findings on ERCP are diagnostic of pancreatitis?** | Beading of the main pancreatic duct with ectatic side branches |
| **What is the medical treatment?** | Alcohol abstinence, analgesics, oral pancreatic enzyme supplements (steatorrhea and malnutrition), and insulin (diabetes) |

## CASE 27

*A 51-year-old female with history of diabetes, obesity, hypertension, and hyperlipidemia complains of stomach pain and pain under the right rib after eating at fast food restaurants. The pain comes on quickly and usually goes away over the next few hours. It does not occur with drinking water or eating fruit. She wonders if she should stop eating at fast food restaurants. Right now, she does not have any pain.*

| | |
|---|---|
| **What is most likely causing her pain?** | Biliary colic from gallstone disease |
| **Why does pain occur is biliary colic?** | The gallbladder contracts after a fatty meal and presses a stone against the gallbladder outlet or cystic duct opening leading to increased pressure within the gallbladder. |
| **What risk factors does she have for gallstones?** | Obesity and diabetes |
| **What are some other risk factors for gallstone formation?** | Crohn disease, cirrhosis, and pregnancy |
| **When should biliary colic be suspected?** | Intermittent right upper quadrant or midepigastric discomfort or pain that may radiate to the back or to the tip of the scapula |
| **What lab tests should be ordered?** | CBC, liver function panel, amylase, lipase, and Chem 8 |

| | |
|---|---|
| **What imaging study should be ordered?** | Right upper quadrant (RUQ) US |
| **How is biliary colic diagnosed?** | History, presentation, and US revealing gallstones |
| **How is biliary colic treated?** | Laparoscopic cholecystectomy |
| **Why is it important to treat it?** | To decrease risk of developing acute cholecystitis |
| **What causes cholecystitis?** | A stone becomes impacted in the cystic duct and inflammation develops behind it (unlike biliary colic where it only intermittently obstructs it). |
| **What triggers it?** | A large or fatty meal just like with biliary colic |
| **How does cholecystitis present?** | Constant severe right upper quadrant pain (may radiate to the right infrascapular area), nausea, vomiting, fever, and leukocytosis |
| **By assessing symptoms, how can you quickly distinguish this from biliary colic?** | The RUQ pain often lasts for more than 4–6 hours, and fever is often present. |
| **What are the common physical exam findings?** | Ill appearing, fever, tachycardia, and lying still because of underlying parietal peritoneal inflammation, voluntary and involuntary guarding |
| **What is a key sign found on physical exam?** | Murphy sign (pain elicited by placing the hand under rib cage on inspiration) |
| **What labs should be ordered?** | Same as in biliary colic |
| **How is acute cholecystitis diagnosed?** | History, presentation, US and/or HIDA (more sensitive), and elevated WBC |
| **What is the treatment for acute cholecystitis?** | NPO, IV fluids, analgesics, and antibiotics followed by laparoscopic cholecystectomy after the patient is stable |

| | |
|---|---|
| **What would you be concerned about if the last patient was jaundiced and had an elevated conjugated bilirubin?** | Acute cholangitis |
| **How does acute cholangitis present?** | Sudden onset of RUQ pain, fever, and jaundice (Charcot triad); nausea and vomiting may also be present. |
| **What commonly causes acute cholangitis?** | Gallstones promote bile stasis and serve as a nidus of infection for bacteria from the duodenum to ascend the biliary tract. |
| **What are the common organisms?** | *Enterococcus, Escherichia coli*, and *Klebsiella* |
| **What lab finding suggests the diagnosis?** | Bilirubinuria, high conjugated bilirubin, and alkaline phosphatase |
| **How is cholangitis diagnosed?** | History, presentation, ERCP (US and HIDA less reliable) |
| **What is the treatment for cholangitis?** | After stabilizing the patient, proceed with endoscopic removal of common bile duct stone with ERCP followed by laparoscopic cholecystectomy. |

## CASE 28

*A 48-year-old male with history of liver cirrhosis secondary to chronic hepatitis C, colon cancer s/p resection 8 years ago with normal colonoscopy report 6 months ago presents to your office with an 8-pound weight loss over the last 6 weeks without change in diet or exercise, right upper quadrant discomfort, and jaundice.*

| | |
|---|---|
| **What is the most likely cause?** | Hepatocellular carcinoma (HCC) |
| **Why?** | Chronic hepatitis C and cirrhosis of the liver are both risk factors for HCC. |

| | |
|---|---|
| **What other risk factors are there for a primary liver cancer?** | Chronic hepatitis B, alcoholic cirrhosis, α-1 antitrypsin deficiency, and hemochromatosis |
| **What is the most common cause of liver cancer?** | Metastatic colon and breast cancer (lung, stomach, kidney, and pancreas less common) |
| **Why is colon cancer less likely in this patient?** | Lack of changes in bowel habits and normal colonoscopy within the last 6 months |
| **How does HCC commonly present?** | Often asymptomatic, but may present with mild to moderate upper abdominal pain, weight loss, early satiety, palpable abdominal mass, worsening ascites, encephalopathy, jaundice, or variceal bleeding |
| **What are the associated lab tests?** | Small elevated alkaline phosphatase, occasionally slight increase in ALT or bilirubin |
| **What imaging studies help make the diagnosis?** | US and CT scan |
| **How is the diagnosis made?** | Needle biopsy, often CT or US guided |
| **What studies and tests are available to monitor cirrhotic patients at risk of hepatoma?** | US or CT and α-feto protein at least yearly |
| **What is the treatment?** | Surgical resection for small solitary hepatoma, supportive otherwise |

## CASE 29

*A 44-year-old female with history of rheumatoid arthritis controlled with immunomodulators, cholecystectomy owing to atypical abdominal pain with elevated alkaline phosphatase and serum bilirubin presents to your office after relocating to the area from another state with severe generalized itching. She has tried over-the-counter benadryl for the itching, but it has not helped. Other than excoriations on her arms and legs from scratching, her exam is normal.*

| | |
|---|---|
| **What is the most likely cause of her itching?** | Primary biliary cirrhosis (PBC) |
| **What are the clues in this patient?** | Female gender, severe generalized pruritis, known autoimmune disease (RA), history of elevated alkaline phosphatase and bilirubin |
| **What else may present as the disease progresses?** | Hepatomegaly, weight loss, and diarrhea |
| **What additional features may present years later?** | Jaundice, dark urine, pale stools, and signs of portal hypertension |
| **What causes PBC?** | A slowly progressive autoimmune disease characterized by destruction of intrahepatic ducts and cholestasis |
| **What other diseases may be evident on physical exam?** | Other autoimmune diseases (scleroderma, Sjogren syndrome, pernicious anemia, thyroid disorders, rheumatoid arthritis, and vitaligo) |
| **What lab test results suggest the diagnosis?** | Increased alkaline phosphatase and bilirubin |
| **What test results are more specific to PBC?** | Positive antimitochondrial antibody and elevated serum IgM levels |
| **How is the diagnosis confirmed?** | Liver biopsy |
| **What medication may delay early-stage disease progression?** | Ursodeoxycholic acid |
| **What medication is used to treat pruritus?** | Cholestyramine |

## CASE 30

*A 35-year-old male with long-standing history of ulcerative colitis follows up in your clinic for his yearly exam after having pre-clinic labs done. His CBC and chemistry panel are normal, but the alkaline phosphatase is elevated 3× the normal value.*

**What disease process are you most concerned about?**

Primary sclerosing cholangitis (PSC)

**Why?**

Ulcerative colitis is a risk factor for PSC.

**What is PSC?**

A chronic cholestatic disease of unknown etiology characterized by diffuse inflammation, fibrosis, and eventual destruction of extrahepatic and intrahepatic bile ducts

**Do the disease activities of PSC and IBD correlate with each other?**

No

**How do most patients present?**

With elevated cholestatic liver function tests, especially alkaline phosphatase

**What symptoms or signs might he have?**

Fatigue and pruritus

**What sign suggests advanced PSC?**

Jaundice

**What noninvasive imaging test can be helpful in making a diagnosis?**

RUQ US or MRI

**Is a liver biopsy required to make the diagnosis?**

No

**How is the diagnosis confirmed?**

ERCP with cholangiogram demonstrating multifocal stricturing and dilation of intrahepatic and/or extrahepatic bile ducts

**What is the treatment?**

ERCP for balloon dilatation of local strictures and liver transplant for end-stage liver disease patients

**Does a colectomy in IBD patients protect against PSC?**

No

**What are PSC patients at increased risk of developing?**

Cholangiocarcinoma

## PANCREAS

### CASE 31

*A 55-year-old businessman with history of HTN, hyperlipidemia, and arthritis presents to the ER Saturday night after entertaining clients at a professional hockey game complaining of severe acute 10/10 epigastric pain that radiates to the back with nausea and nonbloody emesis. This has never occurred before. Lately, his other medical conditions have been well controlled by his primary care doctor. However, he has been urinating more after his doctor put him on a hydrochlorothiazide about a week ago. On physical exam, you detect alcohol on his breath and tenderness to palpation in the epigastric area; otherwise the exam is within normal limits.*

| | |
|---|---|
| **What could be causing his pain?** | Acute pancreatitis, PUD, gastritis, esophagitis, cholecystitis |
| **Which is more likely?** | Acute pancreatitis because the pain radiates to the back |
| **Can PUD do that?** | Yes, if the patient has a penetrating ulcer |
| **Is this patient at risk of ulcer disease?** | Possibly; he has arthritis and may be taking over-the-counter aspirin or other NSAIDS. |
| **Why is PUD less likely in this patient?** | No prior episodes of epigastric pain and the current episode occurred acutely |
| **What is the most likely cause then?** | Acute pancreatitis |
| **What's the basic pathogenesis in acute pancreatitis?** | A sudden nonbacterial inflammation of the pancreas that occurs when pancreatic enzymes escape and digest the pancreas and surrounding tissue |

**Name the two most common causes.**

Gallstones disease and alcoholism

**What are his risk factors for acute pancreatitis?**

Hyperlipidemia, hydrochlorothiazide, and alcohol use

**What other risk factors are there?**

Other drugs (e.g., furosemide, steroids), infections (e.g., mumps), cardiac bypass surgery, tumors, and peptic ulcers

**What two findings on physical exam are unique to acute pancreatitis?**

Cullen sign (periumbilic discoloration) and Grey Turner sign (bluish discoloration in the flank area)

**What abnormal lab values would you expect?**

Increased amylase and lipase

**What 3 radiographic tests are helpful in making the diagnosis?**

Ultrasound, abdominal x-ray, and CT scan of abdomen

**Why is the ultrasound useful?**

It's inexpensive and gives valuable information about the bile duct and gallbladder.

**What are the associated abdominal x-ray findings?**

Sentinel loop (dilated bowel loop near pancreas) or the colon cutoff sign (distended gas in the right colon that stops near the pancreas)

**Why is a CT scan of the abdomen useful?**

Can detect extent of pancreatic inflammation and whether or not any sequelae of pancreatitis have developed

**How is the diagnosis made?**

Presentation and associated lab values (increased amylase and lipase)

**What is the initial treatment?**

NPO, nasogastric suction (if vomiting), IV fluids, Foley catheter, antibiotics (if fever) and analgesics (narcotics), and H2 blockers

| | |
|---|---|
| **If medical therapy fails, what is the next step in management?** | Surgical consult |
| **What prognostic criteria are used to assess mortality risk?** | Ranson's criteria |
| **Define Ranson's criteria during the first 24 hours of admission.** | Age >55 years old, blood glucose >200 mg/dL, serum LDH >350 IU/L, serum AST >250, WBC >16,000/mL |
| **Define Ranson's criteria within 48 hours of admission.** | Hematocrit drops >10%, BUN rises >5 mg/dL, serum calcium <8 mg/dL, PaO$_2$ <60 mm Hg, base deficit <4 mEq/L, fluid sequestration <6 L |
| **How many of Ranson's criteria are needed to indicate poor outcome and increased risk of mortality?** | 3 or more |

## CASE 32

*A 41-year-old female smoker recently diagnosed with diabetes presents to your office with jaundice. Her friends noticed that she started looking more yellow about 10 days ago and has gradually progressed. She notes that her acuchecks for her diabetes have been higher even with taking the recommended dose of her medications. The physical exam is unremarkable except for a small right supraclavicular node and yellow skin. She wants to know if the yellow skin is from the diabetes or recently prescribed medication.*

| | |
|---|---|
| **What do you think she has?** | Pancreatic cancer |
| **What is the most common histologic type?** | Adenocarcinoma (often of ductal origin) |
| **What were the clues?** | Smoker (a risk factor), recent diagnosis of diabetes, supraclavicular node (Virchow node), and painless jaundice |

**What other symptoms might be presented to you?**

Icterus, pancreatitis, abdominal pain that radiates to the back, and weight loss

**What other signs may be found on physical exam?**

Periumbilical node (Sister Mary Joseph's node), Courvoisier gallbladder (distended gallbladder as a result of common bile duct obstruction), and rectal shelf mass (Blumer shelf)

**What do these findings suggest?**

Metastatic disease

**What labs should you order?**

Chem 8, LFT, PT

**What are the associated lab values?**

Hyperglycemia and increased bilirubin, alkaline phosphatase, AST, and ALT if bile duct obstruction occurs; PT may be elevated due to malabsorption of vitamin K-dependent factors (II, VII, IX, X)

**What tumor markers may be elevated?**

CA 19–9 and CEA

**What imaging is useful?**

US (locate site of obstruction), CT (determine extent of disease), and ERCP with brushings (biopsy to confirm diagnosis)

**Once the mass is identified, what's the best diagnostic procedure to order?**

Endoscopic ultrasound with fine needle aspiration

**What is the treatment for localized disease?**

Surgical resection

**What medical therapy may be employed for metastatic disease?**

5-FU

## MISCELLANEOUS DISORDERS

CASE 33

*A 47-year-old obese male with history of HTN and hyperlipidemia presents with 3-month history of infrequent, intermittent left groin bulging which occurs most often when lifting heavy boxes at work or straining when going to the bathroom.*

| | |
|---|---|
| **What do you suspect this patient has?** | Inguinal hernia |
| **What risk factors does he have?** | Obesity and excessive straining |
| **What additional risk factor may be present in other patients for an inguinal hernia?** | Pregnancy, chronic cough, and ascites |
| **How do most inguinal hernias present?** | Often asymptomatic and detected on routine physical exam by detecting a mass or bulge in the inguinal canal as the patient coughs |
| **Your physical exam confirms the findings above. What type of inguinal hernia does he have?** | Reducible |
| **What is a reducible hernia at risk of?** | Incarceration |
| **How would the physical exam change?** | The inguinal bulge would become firm, nonreducible with tenderness to palpation |
| **What are the dreaded complications of incarcerated hernias?** | Strangulation and infarction |
| **How is it diagnosed?** | Physical exam |

**What causes an inguinal hernia?**

Protrusion of intra-abdominal contents through a defect in the abdominal wall

**What treatment should you offer this patient with a reducible hernia?**

Elective surgical repair

**What if it becomes nonre-ducible?**

Immediate surgical repair

# 4     Nephrology

## RENAL FAILURE

### CASE I

*A 68-year-old male with history of dementia, congestive heart failure (CHF), degenerative joint disease (DJD), taking NSAIDS and BPH with an elevated prostate-specific antigen (PSA), presents to the ER from the nursing home with recent onset of worsening mental status and decreased urine output. Due to his confused state, it is difficult to obtain additional history. Routine blood work ordered yesterday from the nursing home is provided, and you see that the serum creatinine has increased to 3 from a prior value of 1.2 6 weeks ago.*

| | |
|---|---|
| **What's his new diagnosis?** | Acute renal failure (ARF) |
| **What 3 broad categories could his ARF be caused from?** | Pre-renal, renal, and post-renal |
| **Give examples of each.** | |
| Pre-renal | Inadequate perfusion (volume depletion, CHF, decreased effective blood volume) |
| Renal | Acute tubular necrosis (ATN), acute interstitial nephritis, acute glomeru-lonephritis |
| Post-renal | Obstruction—bladder outlet or bilateral ureteral |
| **What known risk factors does he have for each group?** | |
| Pre-renal | CHF |
| Renal | NSAID-induced nephrotoxicity |
| Post-renal? | BPH; to rule out prostate cancer (PSA is elevated) |

**What key presenting features in the history would raise your suspicion of:**

**Pre-renal?**

History of cardiac events, hypotension, recent decompensation of CHF, cirrhosis

**Renal?**

Drug history, with attention to potential nephrotoxins, including radiocontrast and over-the-counter meds (especially NSAIDS)

**Post-renal?**

Hematuria, retentive symptoms, flank pain, decreased urine output

**What key physical signs would support**

**Pre-renal cause?**

Rales, gallop, edema, jugular vein distention (JVD) (CHF exacerbation) or orthostatics, dry mucosae, poor skin turgor (volume depletion)

**Obstruction?**

Bladder percussion, distention, or abdominal tenderness (including flank pain), nodular enlarged prostate on rectal exam

**What simple bedside procedure, if positive, would support obstructive cause?**

High post-void residual volume

**How is this test done?**

Patient is asked to urinate, then a straight catheter or bladder scanner (ultrasound) is used to determine residual bladder volume.

**What lab tests are used to narrow the differential?**

Urinalysis, urine Na (UNa) and Cr, serum Na, Cr, and BUN (blood urea nitrogen)

**How would you interpret the following urine sodium values?**

**Low UNa (<20 mEq/L)**

Suggests functional tubules stimulated to retain sodium as seen in pre-renal conditions like CHF

| High UNa in a hypoten-sive patient | Renal failure secondary to failure of the tubules to retain Na despite appropriate stimulus |

**What is FENa and how is it calculated?**

Fractional excretion of sodium is a refinement of UNa, by adjusting for urinary concentration

$$FENa = \frac{(UNa/PNa)}{(UCr/PCr)} \times 100\%$$

**What does a FENa <1% imply?**

Tubular retention of Na in attempt to increase glomerular filtration rate (GFR) in such states of pre-renal failure (e.g., CHF)

**What other lab findings suggest pre-renal azotemia?**

BUN/creatinine >20–40, urinary specific gravity >1.025

**How would you interpret the following urine sediment results?**

    **Bland sediment**

Suggests pre-renal failure or obstruction

    **Granular casts, tubular cells, and casts**

Renal failure secondary to ATN often secondary to medications

    **RBC casts**

Renal failure secondary to glomerulonephritis

    **WBCs and WBC casts, with eosinophils**

Renal failure secondary to acute interstitial nephritis

    **Heme positive, without RBCs**

Renal failure secondary to pigmenturia (hemoglobin or myoglobulin)

**What additional workup should be ordered based on the following urine sediment tests?**

    **RBC casts**

Antistreptolysin O (ASO), antineutrophil cytoplasmic antibody, complements, antinuclear antibody (ANA), hepatitis serologies, and possible renal biopsy

| | |
|---|---|
| **WBCs and WBC casts, with eosinophils (AIN)** | Review medications (including over-the-counter and herbal) |
| **Bland sediment not in a pre-renal setting** | Abdominal ultrasound to rule out obstruction (95% sensitive) |

**Describe the appropriate treatment based on cause of ARF.**

| | |
|---|---|
| Pre-renal | Ensure adequate volume, maximize cardiac output |
| **Obstruction** | Relieve obstruction with Foley, percutaneous nephrostomy, etc., as indicated |
| **Acute glomerular nephritis (GN) and rapidly progressive glomerular nephritis (RPGN)** | See sections on those diagnoses. |
| **Acute interstitial nephritis** | Remove offending agents, consider steroids |
| **ATN** | Optimize cardiac output and volume status; loop diuretics to convert oliguric to nonoliguric ATN, if possible; restrict Na, K, protein; dose adjust meds for impaired GFR; avoid further nephrotoxin exposure; dialysis as indicated. |
| **What are the indications for dialysis?** | Volume overload, hyperkalemia, acidosis refractory to medical measures, uremic platelet dysfunction with bleeding, uremic syndrome (encephalopathy, pericarditis) |

## CASE 2

*55-year-old male with history of chronic obstructive pulmonary disease (COPD), multifocal tachycardia, arthritis, hypertension, diabetes, and chronic renal insufficiency presents to your clinic for a routine checkup after obtaining a CBC and CMP. His Cr has increased from 2.5 to 3, Hg is 9.5, HgA1C is 8, $PO_4$ of 6.0, $HCO_3$ of 16.*

**What is the most likely explanation for the following?**

**Increased Cr**

Uncontrolled hypertension or diabetes (the two most common causes of CRF) worsening his underlying CRF

**Elevated HgA1C**

Uncontrolled diabetes

**Low Hg**

Low erythropoietin level secondary to decreased production from failing kidneys

**High PO$_4$**

Secondary to markedly increased parathyroid hormone in CRF patients as an adaptive response in an attempt to maintain normocalcemia

**What should be the goals of this office visit?**

Aggressive BP control, optimize diabetes control, lower PO$_4$, raise Hg

**What's a reasonable approach to the following problems?**

**Elevated BP**

ACE inhibitor (has been shown to decrease risk of progression and development of proteinuria)

**Hg 9.5 (anemia)**

After other factors (vitamin deficiencies, bone marrow disorders) have been excluded, therapy with recombinant human erythropoietin

**High PO$_4$ (secondary hyperparathyroidism)**

Limit dietary phosphate; add a phosphate binder such as calcium acetate or sevelamer to keep PO$_4$ below 5.5 mg/dL; add active vitamin D analogues (calcitriol, doxercalciferol) to lower iPTH

**HCO$_3$ of 16 (chronic metabolic acidosis)**

NaHCO$_3$ given at 650 mg TID to start to maintain serum HCO$_3$ in the 18–20 mEq/L range

**What drugs should be avoided in CRF?**

Nephrotoxins (such as radiocontrast, aminoglycosides) or drugs with significant renal effects (e.g., NSAIDs). Drugs with renal excretion need dose adjustment, as do drugs whose metabolites are renally excreted (e.g., procainamide). Some drugs are avoided entirely (e.g., meperidine).

**Name some indications to start dialysis.**

GFR of 5–10 cc/min/1.73m$^2$ BSA; uremic signs or symptoms start, hyperkalemia, volume overload, acidosis or hypertension refractory to medical measures

**How is GFR calculated?**

$$C_{Creat} = \frac{(140-age) \times \text{lean body mass [kg]}}{72 \times \text{serum creatinine}}$$
$$\times 0.85 \text{ for females}$$

**What are the symptoms of uremia?**

Fatigue, anorexia, metallic or ammoniacal taste, sleep cycle disturbances, pruritis, dyspnoea

**What are the signs of uremia?**

Asterixis, peripheral neuropathy, serositis (especially pericarditis), dry skin, prurigo, signs of volume overload

## FLUID AND ELECTROLYTES

### CASE 3

*A 55-year-old asymptomatic male with history of HTN, hyperlipidemia, diabetes, and DJD comes to your office for a routine office visit after obtaining routine blood tests prior to his visit. His serum chemistry panel is all within normal limits except for his serum Na, which is low at 131.*

**What can you infer from his asymptomatic state?**

The hyponatremia developed slowly. More rapid or severe hyponatremia can cause headache, lassitude, seizure, and coma.

**What four broad groups can hyponatremia be classified into?**

Pseudohyponatremia, hypovolemia, euvolemia, and hypervolemia

**What's the first step in the workup?**

Rule out pseudohyponatremia

**What is pseudohyponatremia?**

Apparent hyponatremia with normal or high serum osmolality caused by severe hyperglycemia, hyperlipidemia (>1200 mg/mL), or severe hyperproteinemia (e.g., myeloma)

**Is he at risk of this?**

Yes, he is a known diabetic and has hyperlipidemia.

**What would you order to rule this out?**

Serum protein, cholesterol, and glucose level (or acucheck).

**What is the therapy for pseudohyponatremia?**

Treat the underlying disorder

**What's the next step if pseudohyponatremia is ruled out?**

Assess volume status (hyper- , hypo- , or euvolemic) on physical exam

**What are some physical exam clues for**

**Hypervolemia?**

Rales, LE edema, JVD (CHF), abdominal ascites (cirrhosis)

**Hypovolemia?**

Orthostatic hypotension, poor skin turgor, dry mucus membranes

**What tests do you order after you establish the patient's volume status?**

Urine Na and urine osmolality

**For each of the conditions below give a brief differential:**

**Hypovolemic hyponatremia with UNa >20**

Renal loses by diuretics, hypoaldosteronism, or salt-wasting nephropathy

**Hypovolemic hyponatremia with UNa <10**

Extra-renal losses through GI tract, third spacing or insensible losses

**Euvolemic hyponatremia with urine osmolality <100**

Psychogenic polydipsia (drinking excessive quantities of water)

**Euvolemic hyponatremia with urine osmolality >100**

SIADH

**Hypervolemic hypona-tremia and UNa <10**

CHF, cirrhosis, or nephrotic syndrome

**Hypervolemic hypona-tremia and UNa >20**

Renal failure

**Why is volume overload (CHF, cirrhosis, nephrosis) commonly associated with hyponatremia?**

Despite pathologic sodium retention, even greater amounts of water have been retained, resulting in a dilution of the excess sodium, hence the term "dilutional hyponatremia" often applied here. CHF and decreased *effective* plasma volume stimulate ADH, causing water retention. The renal diluting mechanism may be impaired, due to decreased GFR and distal Na delivery. In hospitals, sodium restriction is enforced more successfully than free water restriction.

**What is SIADH?**

Normovolemic hyponatremia (i.e., net free water accumulation) in a patient lacking known pathophysiologic stimuli to ADH release, such as CHF, cirrhosis, pain, and nausea. Must rule out endocrine disorders (thyroid, adrenal). Urine shows ADH effect: less than maximally dilute.

**What is SIADH usually associated with?**

(1) Intrathoracic processes: lung cancer (primary or metastatic to lung), bronchiec-tasis, tuberculosis

(2) Intracranial events: hemorrhage, meningitis, encephalitis, tumors

**What drugs may produce an SIADH-like picture?**

Chlorpropamide, narcotics, phenoth-iazines, tricyclics, SSRIs, carbamezpine, vincristine cytoxan, clofibrate. NSAIDs potentiate ADH effect.

**How is hypovolemic hyponatremia treated?**

Volume replacement with saline, monitor serum sodium

**How is SIADH treated?**

Fluid restriction is key, but often difficult to achieve. High protein intake may be helpful, by increasing daily osmotic load to be excreted. Demeclocycline, to deliberately produce nephrogenic DI, has been used in difficult cases. Very low Na (120 mEq/L or less) requires ICU for administration of 3% hypertonic saline.

**How is hypervolemic hyponatremia treated?**

Fluid restriction is vital. Treat underlying disease (CHF, cirrhosis), and administer diuretics, with careful monitoring of electrolytes.

**What are the risks of over-rapid correction of hyponatremia?**

Central pontine myelinosis may occur if rate of correction is greater than 1–2 mEq/L/hour, or if total increase is over 25 mEq/L over 48 hours. In mild, less symptomatic cases, the correction should be limited to 0.5 mEq/L/hour, or 12 mEq/24 hours.

## CASE 4

*A 48-year-old female with history of menorrhagia post-op day 2 after hysterectomy for uterine fibroids is found to have an elevated serum Na at 156 on am labs.*

**What symptoms of hypernatremia may be present?**

Depending on severity and rapidity of rise, may see irritability, nausea, confusion, obtundation, fasciculations, seizures

**When are symptoms more likely to occur?**

Severe elevation or rapid increase from prior baseline serum Na level

**What should be done first on physical exam to work up the elevated Na?**

Assess volume status (vital signs, orthostatics, rales, edema, skin turgor, mucus membranes)

**What typically causes hypernatremia and volume overload?**

Excess administration of normal saline or sodium bicarbonate; usually occurs in hospital

**If the patient is diagnosed to be hypovolemic or euvolemic, what lab test should be ordered next to narrow your differential?**

Urine osmolality

**What's a reasonable differential for the following urine osmolality?**

**<300**

Complete diabetes insipidus (DI)

**300–600**

Renal water loss (diuretics or osmotic diuresis with glucose urea or mannitol), partial DI, reset osmostat

**>600**

Extra-renal water losses (GI or insensible losses)

**What is central diabetes insipidus?**

Inability of the pituitary to respond normally to hypertonicity by releasing ADH. This may be a complete or partial lack of ADH release.

**What are the causes?**

Idiopathic, seen in childhood. Adult cases are usually due to head trauma, tumors, or encephalitis.

**What is nephrogenic diabetes insipidus?**

Lack of response of concentrating segment of collecting tubules to ADH. This may also be partial or complete.

**What are the causes?**

In adults, hypercalcemia, toxins (e.g., lithium, demeclocycline), hypokalemia, obstructive nephropathy. May be congenital in children. Tubulointerstitial nephritis may reduce the corticomedullary gradient, thereby impairing the concentrating mechanism, but not to the degree seen in true nephrogenic DI.

| | |
|---|---|
| **How is diagnosis of diabetes insipidus confirmed?** | Water deprivation test, with administration of aqueous pitressin to differentiate central from nephrogenic DI |
| **What is the treatment?** | Volume depletion, excess treated in usual manner with saline, diuretics, respectively. Calculate free water deficit = $0.6 \times weight(lean) \times [(Na - 140)/140]$. Replace with D5W slowly, to lower Na by $1$–$2$ mEq/L/hour. |
| **How is central DI treated?** | With ADH or synthetic ADH analogues, such as DDAVP. Ensure adequate access to free water. |
| **How is nephrogenic DI treated?** | Paradoxically, thiazides reduce urine output by blocking the tubular diluting segment. This works best with moderate Na restriction. Ensure free water access. NSAIDs and amiloride may also be of use in reducing urine output, the latter in cases due to chronic lithium use. |

## CASE 5

*A 44-year-old previously healthy male returns to your clinic 1 week after presenting to your clinic for the first time complaining of generalized weakness. No significant findings were found on physical exam and the patient denied symptoms of depression or insomnia. You obtained a comprehensive metabolic panel, CBC, and TSH level. All the results are within normal limits except for the potassium level, which is 3.0.*

| | |
|---|---|
| **Could this explain his generalized weakness?** | Yes, weakness is one of the manifestations of hypokalemia. |
| **What are some other typical clinical manifestations of hypokalemia?** | Muscle cramps, paralytic ileus, cardiac arrhythmias and digtoxicity, glucose intolerance, polyuria |
| **What are typical EKG changes in hypokalemia?** | Lowering of T wave height and appearance of U waves |

**His EKG is normal and you've begun to supplement his potassium. What's the first step in working up his hypokalemia?**

Check a urine potassium level

**What's your differential if the urine K is <25 mEq/d or <15 mEq/L?**

GI losses such as in diarrhea, laxative abuse, vomiting, or NG suction losses

**What's your differential if the Urine K is >30 mEq or >15 mEq/L?**

Renal losses

**What's the next step when hypokalemia is secondary to renal loss?**

Check BP to assess if patient is hypertensive, normotensive, or hypotensive

**What type of potassium wasting diseases need to be considered if the patient is hypertensive?**

Primary (Conn syndrome) or secondary hyperaldosteronism (renal artery stenosis or renin-secreting tumors), and pseudohyperaldosteronism (Cushing syndrome)

**What's the next step for patients whose blood pressure is normal or low?**

Assess acid–base status

**What the differential for the following acid–base states?**
    **Acidemic**

Diabetic ketoacidosis or renal tubular acidosis (RTA)

    **Alkalemic**

Diuretics; vomiting or NG suction; Bartter or Gitelman's disease

**What's the treatment strategy for hypokalemia?**

Supplement potassium and Mg as necessary; treat underlying cause; repeat potassium level after supplementation

**For each 1 mEq/L deficit, how much total body potassium needs to be replaced?**

200 mEq

| | |
|---|---|
| **What's a standard oral dosing regimen for potassium supplementation in nonurgent cases?** | KCl 40 mEq PO q 4–6 hours |
| **Is there any role for K-sparing diuretics?** | Yes, these are useful in chronic situations provided the patient's K can be adequately monitored. Spironolactone is of particular value in cases of secondary hyperaldosteronism, e.g., cirrhosis and CHF. |

## CASE 6

*A 54-year-old male is seen in the ER for epigastric pain felt secondary to peptic ulcer disease as a result of his significant intake of ibuprofen over the last 2 weeks for arthritic pain. Because he has a normal hemoglobin value, and no nausea, vomiting, or blood per rectum, you are preparing to discharge the patient on protonix (a proton pump inhibitor to decrease gastric acid) and follow up with his primary care physician when his serum chemistry comes back. His K is elevated at 6.2.*

| | |
|---|---|
| **What's the revised diagnosis?** | Hyperkalemia |
| **Above what value is hyperkalemia defined?** | >5.2 mEq/L |
| **What symptom of hyperkalemia might he describe?** | Weakness |
| **What should you do first?** | Rule out lab error by repeating test and obtain an EKG. |
| **What can cause lab error (pseudohyperkalemia)?** | High potassium readings in blood specimens that do not reflect the true potassium level *in vivo*. This may be seen in thrombocytosis, due to release of platelet K in the clot formed in a red-top tube; difficult venipuncture or hemolysis. |

**What EKG findings of hyper-kalemia will you look for?**

At first, peaked T waves, with a short QT interval, followed by widened QRS complexes and loss of the P wave, culminating in a "sine wave" pattern which leads rapidly to ventricular fibrillation or asystole. This progression may proceed rapidly.

**If hyperkalemia is confirmed, what's your approach?**

Treat the hyperkalemia first then proceed with your workup.

**What's the treatment for asymptomatic (no EKG changes) patients?**

5–10 units of insulin and 25–50 cc D50 glucose (shifts K into cells) and 30–60 g of Kayexalate by mouth (promotes GI loss of K). Hemodialysis is effective in cases of renal failure.

**What additional therapy is needed if EKG changes are present?**

Calcium gluconate 10% 10 cc, repeat as needed to reverse EKG changes. This does **not** lower serum K, it stabilizes the myocardium and counters arrhythmias.

**What can cause hyperkalemia (not pseudohyperkalemia)?**

Excessive potassium intake, decreased renal excretion, redistribution

**Give some common examples of each.**

**Excessive potassium intake**

Potassium replacement therapy, high-potassium diet

**Decreased renal excretion**

Potassium-sparing diuretics (e.g., spironolactone, triamterene, amiloride), renal insufficiency, Type 4 RTA, ACE inhibitors, heparin, NSAIDs, β-blockers

**Redistribution (excessive cellular release)**

Insulin deficiency, hemolysis, tissue necrosis, rhabdomyolysis, and burns

**What's the mechanism of hyperkalemia in the following medications?**

**β-blockers**

Inhibits renin release and blocks cellular uptake of K if nonselective

| | |
|---|---|
| **ACE inhibitors** | Blocks angiotensin II production |
| **Angiotensin receptor blockers and spironolactone?** | Inhibits aldosterone |
| **Heparin** | Blocks adrenal synthesis of aldosterone |
| **NSAIDs** | Reduces renin release |
| **Amiloride and triamterene** | Blocks renal K excretion |
| **Once redistribution has been ruled out as a cause, what test should be ordered next?** | Transtubular K gradient (TTKG) |

**What is TTKG?**

The TTKG is given by the formula

$$\{U_K/(U_{osm}/P_{osm})\}/P_K$$

It estimates what the urine-to-plasma K gradient would be at the end of the distal tubule, prior to the concentrating segments of the nephron, and as such corrects for the effects of urinary concentration on interpreting urinary K.

**How is it useful?**

A normal value is 6–9; a lower value in hyperkalemia suggests hypoaldosteronism or impaired renal response to aldosterone.

**What is Type IV RTA?**

Hyperkalemia with inadequate renal K excretion despite only mild to moderate CRF, also called tubular hyperkalemia, overlaps with hyporeninemic hypoaldosteronism. Seen in diabetes, chronic interstitial nephritis, systemic lupus erythematosus (SLE), sickle cell disease, obstructive uropathy. May be due to combination of low renin production, reduced aldosterone synthesis, and impaired tubular response to aldosterone; the latter cause is most common.

## GLOMERULAR DISEASES

### CASE 7

*A 12-year-old girl presents to the clinic with new onset of hypertension, peripheral edema, joint pain, and dark urine over the last few days. Recently she had a sore throat for which she was given some over-the-counter herbal remedy and Tylenol.*

| | |
|---|---|
| **What do you suspect?** | Nephritic syndrome secondary to post group A β-hemolytic *Streptococcus* infection |
| **What's the differential for nephritic syndrome?** | Post group A β-hemolytic *Streptococcus* infection, SLE, vasculitis (Wegener granulomatosis, polyarteritis nodosa), idiopathic glomerulonephritis (membranoproliferative, idiopathic, crescentic, IgA nephropathy), Goodpasture syndrome, Henoch-Schönlein purpura |
| **What is nephritic syndrome?** | Acute or subacute glomerulonephritis manifesting with hematuria and red blood cell casts |
| **Why do you suspect post-streptococcal GN (PSGN) in this patient?** | Sore-throat preceded nephritis signs |
| **What usually causes PSGN?** | Nephritogenic strains of group A β-hemolytic *Streptococcus*. The infection may be pharyngitis, or, more commonly worldwide, impetigo. |
| **Describe the classic presenting features in** | |
| **PSGN** | Gross hematuria (described as "Coca-Cola urine"), edema, hypertension |
| **Goodpasture syndrome** | Acute GN signs and pulmonary involvement, often with frank hemoptysis |

| | |
|---|---|
| **Wegener granulomatosis** | Epistaxis and sinusitis are common presentations in addition to neprhtitic signs |
| **IgA nephropathy (also known as Berger disease)** | Male with loin pain and gross hematuria shortly after pharyngitis (viral), with spontaneous resolution until the next episode |
| **Henoch-Schönlein purpura (HSP)** | Palpable purpura and GI involvement |
| **What physical exam finding may be found in patients with nephritic syndrome?** | Hypertension, edema (peripheral, periorbital, or pulmonary), joint pains, dark urine, malar rash (in SLE), palpable purpura (in patients with HSP), heart murmurs (suspect endocarditis), pharyngeal erythema (group A β-hemolytic *Streptococcus* infection) |
| **What initial labs should be ordered to confirm nephritis syndrome?** | Urinalysis, serum creatinine, BUN, 24-hour urine for protein excretion and creatinine clearance |
| **What results are consistent with GN?** **Urinalysis** | Hematuria (dysmorphic erythrocytes and red cell casts) and proteinuria |
| **24-hour urine for protein excretion** | 500 mg/day to 3 g/day |
| **Are RBC casts pathognomonic of GN?** | No. They may be seen in acute interstitial nephritis and, rarely, after vigorous exercise. In the correct clinical setting, however, they are very strong evidence for GN. |
| **Are RBC casts always seen in GN?** | No. After formation in the tubular lumen, they degenerate fairly quickly, forming pigmented coarse granular casts. RBC casts are always accompanied by free RBCs, which, to the trained observer, are dysmorphic, suggesting glomerular origin. Often, several urine specimens need to be examined to demonstrate RBC casts. |

**What additional tests should be ordered if the following is suspected as the cause of the GN?**

| | |
|---|---|
| **PSGN** | Streptococcal tests (Streptozyme), ASO quantitative titer |
| **SLE** | Anti-DNA antibodies |
| **Wegener granulomatosis** | c-ANCA |
| **Paucimmune RPGN (Wegener disease, Churg-Strauss disease, and microscopic polyarteritis nodosa)** | P-ANCA |
| **Goodpasture syndrome** | Anti-GBM antibody |
| **IgA nephropathy (a.k.a. Berger disease)** | Serum IgA level |

**What utility does renal ultrasound have in the workup?**
Estimates kidney size, which helps distinguish between acute and chronic renal disease

**What's the general acute treatment for nephritic syndrome?**
Correction of electrolyte abnormalities and acidosis if present. Treat hypertension with furosemide, hydralazine, or nifedipine.

**What additional treatment is recommended for**

**PSGN?**
Treatment of streptococcal infection with penicillin (or erythromycin in penicillin-allergic patients)

**Goodpasture syndrome?**
Plasmapheresis, followed by prednisone and cyclophosphamide

**Wegener granulomatosis?**
Steroids and cyclophosphamide. Plasmapheresis is not well established here.

| **IgA nephropathy?** | ACE inhibitors and fish oil. Steroids and cytotoxic agents are reserved for cases with nephrotic syndrome and/or progressive azotemia. |
|---|---|
| **P-ANCA positive RPGN?** | Pulse methylprednisolone (often with cyclophosphamide or azathioprine) |

## CASE 8

*A 44-year-old with diabetic retinopathy and neuropathy calls your office while you are on-call complaining of ankle swelling and puffiness around the eyes. She denies chest pain, abdominal swelling, or shortness of breath with exertion.*

| **What known complication of diabetes should you be concerned about in this patient?** | Nephrotic syndrome |
|---|---|
| **What other prior complication of diabetes does she have that is almost always associated with nephritic syndrome?** | Retinopathy |
| **What are some of the symptoms of nephrotic syndrome?** | Swelling, foaming of the urine. Nonspecific findings may include fatigue. The underlying illness (e.g., DM, SLE) may produce additional symptoms. |
| **What are commons signs of nephrotic syndrome?** | The hallmark sign is edema, which may just be dependent (ankles at the end of the day) or generalized anasarca, including periorbital edema. Ascites and pleural effusions may be present. Additional signs may be present attributable to the underlying disorder. |
| **What are the known primary and secondary causes of nephritic syndrome?** | |
| Primary | Focal segmental glomerulosclerosis, membranous nephropathy, minimal change disease, membroproliferative glomerulonephritis, and IgA nephropathy |

| | |
|---|---|
| **Secondary** | Diabetes, SLE, amyloid, drugs/toxins (penicillamine, gold, NSAIDs, heroin, ACEI), infections (HBV, HCV, syphilis), malignancy |
| **Is there a unifying mechanism leading to these phenomena?** | The loss of albumin through the pathologically leaky glomerular basement membrane leads to hypoalbuminemia. The resulting fall in plasma oncotic pressure leads to increased hepatic synthesis of cholesterol, sodium retention by the kidneys, and the development of edema. The kidneys also lose other proteins such as opsonins, and clotting factors. |
| **What's the basic workup?** | Spot urine for protein and urine sediment, 24-hour protein, serum albumin, glucose |
| **What results do you expect for** | |
| **Urinalysis?** | Elevated protein |
| **Urine sediment?** | Oval fat bodies, free fat droplets, and fatty casts. Refractile bodies (Maltese cross appearance) may be seen. The sediment *may* also contain nephritic (q.v.) elements. |
| **Serum protein?** | <3 g/dL |
| **24-hour urine protein?** | At least 3.5 g/24 hours (confirms nephritic syndrome) |
| **What additional lab test should be ordered in a diabetic?** | HgA1c (assess diabetic control over last 3 months) |
| **What additional tests should be ordered when the cause is unclear (not diabetes or drug/toxin related)?** | ANA, SPEP (if suspect myeloma), compliment (C3, C4, CH-50), LDH, hepatitis B and C screening, and HIV |
| **What's the final step in the workup?** | Renal biopsy (confirms the diagnosis) |

| **What is the general therapy?** | Avoidance of nephrotoxic drugs and treat underlying secondary cause if found, Na restriction and diuretics for edema, support hose for legs |
|---|---|
| **What medication should be considered to decrease proteinuria and progression to ESRD in diabetic and nondiabetic nephropathy with moderate to severe proteinuria?** | ACE inhibitor |
| **What therapy may be considered for primary glomerular disease?** | Steroids and cytotoxic therapy (e.g., cyclophosphamide, chlorambucil) |

## FLANK PAIN

### CASE 9

*A 32-year-old previously healthy female presents to your clinic complaining of nausea, vomiting, dysuria, and sudden onset of severe flank pain.*

| **What's your differential diagnosis?** | Urinary tract infection, nephrolithiasis, pyelonephritis, diverticulitis, PID, ovarian pathology, appendicitis, small bowel obstruction, ectopic pregnancy |
|---|---|
| **Further questioning reveals that the pain radiates to the groin. What's the most likely diagnosis?** | Nephrolithiasis |
| **How does the stone patient typically present?** | With renal colic, characterized by severe, intermittent, unilateral flank pain lasting 20–60 minutes that radiates to the groin or testicle; dysuria, frequency, nausea, vomiting, and gross hematuria may also be present |

**Name the 4 major types of kidney stones.**

Calcium oxalate, uric acid, struvite, and cystine.

**What is the most common type?**

Calcium oxalate

**What endocrine disorder is a risk factor for developing calcium oxalate stones?**

Hyperparathyroidism

**Which type of stone is associated with urea-splitting bacteria (*Pseudomonas*, *Proteus*, *Klebsiella*) and high urinary pH?**

Struvite

**What basic diagnostic tests are included in the workup?**

Urinalysis, BUN, creatinine, serum calcium, KUB x-ray, and CBC (if febrile). Further metabolic workup, including urine collections, are deferred until patient has recovered from acute episode and has returned to usual diet.

**What type of stone is not seen on x-ray?**

Uric acid stones

**What additional diagnostic test may be ordered if suspicion is high in patient with normal renal function and KUB?**

Intravenous pyelogram, which has been the gold standard, although CTT scanning may replace it

**What test may be useful if obstruction is suspected?**

Renal ultrasound, which may also detect radiolucent stones missed on KUB

**What is the treatment?**

Hydration (oral or IV) and analgesics (narcotics or NSAIDs) as needed for pain

**What additional treatment is required if infection is present?**

IV antibiotics and aggressive workup for obstruction

**What treatment should be considered if an upper tract stone does not pass?**

Extracorporeal shock wave lithotripsy to break up stone into smaller fragments which will then be able to pass

**What treatment may be useful if stone is located in the lower urinary tract?**

Surgical extraction per cystoscopy

## CASE 10

*A 78-year-old nursing home patient with history of dementia, DJD, and urinary incontinence with an indwelling Foley catheter presents to the ER with an acute worsening of her mental status, fever of 103°F, chills, nausea, vomiting, and complaints of severe right flank pain.*

**What diagnosis do you suspect?**

Pyelonephritis with likely urosepsis

**What major risk factor did this patient have for pyelonephritis?**

Indwelling catheter

**What other risk factors for pyelonephritis are there?**

Urinary tract obstruction, stasis, diabetes mellitus, immunocompromised state, and nephrolithiasis

**Does pyelonephritis commonly present like this?**

Yes, it often presents with sudden onset of fever, chills, nausea, vomiting, and flank pain with or without concomitant UTI symptoms

**What physical exam finding would support your diagnosis?**

Right costovertebral tenderness

**What labs should you order and why?**

UA with culture and sensitivity (confirm infection), blood cultures (assess for bacteremia and aid in future antibiotic selection), CBC with differential (to rule out leukocytosis), Chem 8 (to rule out dehydrated or electrolyte abnormalities)

**Can you get the UA from the indwelling Foley?**

No, it will be colonized with bacteria; a straight catheter specimen or clean catch specimen must be obtained.

**What results do you suspect in the**

    **UA?**  Elevated leukocyte esterase, nitrates, and WBC casts in the urinalysis

    **Blood cultures?**  Gram-negative rods

**Lab tests come back positive for UTI and GNR bacteremia. What noninvasive test can aid in diagnosing pyelonephritis?**  Renal ultrasound

**Renal ultrasound is positive for right ureter and calyx dilatation consistent with pyelonephritis. What's your diagnosis?**  Urosepsis secondary to pyelonephritis secondary to UTI from indwelling catheter (possibly partially obstructed)

**Which GNR do you suspect?**  *E. coli* (often ascends from the lower urinary tract)

**What is the treatment?**  Remove indwelling catheter, IV fluoroquinolone (ciprofloxacin) or third-generation cephalosporin (ceftriaxone) for 1 to 2 days followed by oral ciprofloxacin for 2 weeks

## MISCELLANEOUS DISORDERS

CASE 11

*A 57-year-old previously healthy male presents with insidious onset of difficulty with urination. He states it is difficult to start urinating and has taken progressively longer to drain his bladder. At first, it was not bothersome, but now he is going to the bathroom twice as often.*

**What's your differential diagnosis?**  Benign prostatic hypertrophy (BPH), diabetes, urologic cancer, calculi, UTI, stricture disease, and a neurologic disorder

**Which do you suspect?**  BPH

| | |
|---|---|
| **Why?** | BPH often presents with urinary obstruction symptoms (hesitancy, decreased stream strength, dribbling, urinary retention, and sense of incomplete emptying). |
| **What causes BPH?** | A benign adenomatous hyperplasia of the prostate gland which compresses the prostatic urethra resulting in decreased urine flow |
| **What physical exam finding would support your suspicion?** | An enlarged prostate |
| **What lab tests should you order and why?** | UA (UTI?), Blood urea nitrogen/ Creatinine ratio (BUN/Cr) (renal failure?), PSA (prostate cancer?), post-void residual volume (overdistended bladder?) |
| **Enlarged prostate is found on PE and above labs are normal. Do you still suspect BPH?** | Yes |
| **What diagnostic test can you order to confirm your diagnosis?** | Transrectal ultrasound (increased sensitivity) |
| **What is the initial treatment?** | α-blockers (e.g., prazosin, terazosin) to inhibit urinary bladder sphincter contractions and hormone therapy (5-α reductase) to inhibit prostatic conversion of testosterone to dihydrotestosterone which reduces prostate size |
| **What is the next step if medical intervention fails?** | Surgery with transurethral prostatectomy |

## CASE 12

*A 37-year-old obese diabetic female at 30 weeks gestation presents to the office complaining of burning on urination.*

| | |
|---|---|
| **What's your differential diagnosis?** | UTI, vaginitis, pyelonephritis |
| **Which is most likely?** | UTI |
| **Why are the following less likely?** | |
| **Vaginitis** | Often has vaginal discharge |
| **Pyelonephritis** | No fever, nausea, vomiting, chills, elevated temperature, or CVA tenderness |
| **What additional questions would you want to ask to support a diagnosis of UTI?** | Any increased urinary frequency, urgency, nocturia, suprapubic pain, hematuria, or history of UTI |
| **What risk factors does she have for a UTI?** | DM and pregnancy |
| **Name other UTI risk factors** | Recent sexual activity (worth asking about), congenital urologic abnormalities, immunocompromised states |
| **Who is at greatest risk of UTIs?** | Sexually active women |
| **What physical exam signs of UTI may be present?** | Suprapubic pain (common) and fever (uncommon) |
| **What's the workup?** | |
| **First-line test** | UA |
| **What values are diagnostic of a UTI?** | Positive leukocyte esterase, increased nitrates, increased pH |
| **What is the next test if the UA is positive?** | Urine culture with sensitivities |
| **What bacterial count is diagnostic of a UTI?** | A single species with >100,000 bacteria/mL |
| **Which Gram stain finding and organism are most common?** | Gram-negative bacteria, *E. coli* |

**What's the treatment?**
    **First-line**                       A 3–7 day oral course of trimethoprim-
                                         sulfamethoxazole

    **If sulfa allergy?**                Amoxacillin or ciprofloxacin

CASE 13

*An 18-year-old female with history of UTIs, cervical HPV, drug abuse, and 2 prior abortions presents to your office complaining of painful urination and purulent vaginal discharge.*

**What's your differential diagnosis?**                     UTI, urethritis, candidiasis

**What diagnosis do you suspect?**                          Urethritis

**Why?**                                                    Vaginal discharge is common in urethritis and patient has risk factors for it [multiple sexual partners, UTIs, drug abuse, and STDs (cervical HPV)]

**What two organisms cause urethritis in women?**           Gonococcal (GC) or nongonococcal (NGC)

**What symptoms may occur in both?**                        UTI symptoms (increased frequency, urgency, and dysuria)

**Which infectious organism is most likely in this patient?**   GC urethritis because the discharge is purulent (NGC is often described as thin, clear to white scanty discharge)

**What lab tests should you order?**                        UA, culture and Gram stain of urethral discharge (or cervical mucus in women)

**What's your diagnosis if the lab reports**
    **Gram-negative intracellular diplococci in WBCs or positive Thayer-Martin culture?**     GC urethritis

    **Negative Gram stain?**                                NGC urethritis

**What causes GC urethritis?**  *Neisseria gonorrhoeae*

**What causes NGC urethritis?**  *Chlamydia trachomatis* and ureaplasma urealyticum

**Ironically, what is the treatment strategy?**  Treat both GC and NGC because of high incidence of co-infection

**So, what is the treatment?**  Ceftrixone (for GC) and doxycycline, tertracycline, or zithromax (for NGC)

**What are patients at risk for without treatment?**  Urinary strictures, PID, and infertility

# 5    Endocrine Disorders

## DIABETES MELLITUS

### CASE I

*A 12-year-old female presents to her physician with her mother after abnormal behavior concerning for anorexia. The mother states that over the last 2 weeks her daughter has lost weight while eating and drinking more than usual and she goes to the bathroom frequently. The mother, a recovering anorexic herself, is worried her daughter has the disease. The daughter says she feels fine, but has noticed her vision is blurred once and a while.*

| | |
|---|---|
| **What's your differential diagnosis?** | Diabetes insipidus, diabetes mellitus, stress hyperglycemia, diabetes secondary to hormonal excess, drugs, pancreatic disease, anorexia |
| **What are you most concerned about?** | Diabetes mellitus (DM) |
| **Why?** | Age under 30 with an abrupt onset of weight loss, polydipsia, polyphagia, and polyuria is most concerning for diabetes mellitus. |
| **Which type?** | Type 1 |
| **What are other names for it?** | Insulin-dependent diabetes mellitus and juvenile onset diabetes |
| **What's the mechanism of type 1 diabetes?** | Hyperglycemia secondary to relative or complete lack of insulin secretion by the β cells of the pancreas |
| **What damages the insulin receptors?** | Islet cell antibodies (found in 90% of patients within the first year of diagnosis) and viral infections (mumps and Coxsackie virus) have been suggested. |

| | |
|---|---|
| **What basic labs should you order?** | Chem 8 (assess electrolytes, dehydration, kidney function, and glucose level) |
| **How is it diagnosed in** **Asymptomatic patients?** | Either by a fasting plasma glucose greater than 126 mg/dL on two separate occasions or by a positive 2-hour oral glucose tolerance test (2 values at 2 hours exceed 200 mg/dL) |
| **Symptomatic patients?** | Presence of symptoms (weight loss, polyuria, etc.) with a random plasma glucose greater than 200 mg/dL |
| **What is the initial treatment?** | Diabetic diet (60% carbohydrates, 15% protein, and 25% fat not exceeding 35 kcal/kg/day) and physical activity to attain ideal body weight |
| **How is the DM monitored?** | Numerous daily capillary blood glucose measurements |
| **What are the recommended fasting, preprandial, and postprandial glucose levels?** | Fasting and preprandial between 70 and 120 mg/dL and postprandial less than 160 mg/dL |
| **What lab test is used to assess glycemic control over the last 4 weeks?** | Glycosylated hemoglobin $A_1C$ |
| **What is the next therapy in type 1 DM?** | Insulin |
| **What chronic conditions are they at risk of with poor disease management?** | Signs of end-organ complications (retinopathy, neuropathy, peripheral vascular disease, macrovascular disease, nephropathy, foot disease, and depression) |

## CASE 2

*A 45-year-old female with history of hypertension, obesity, and recently diagnosed hyperlipidemia visits your office 6 weeks after starting her lipid-lowering medication after failing diet and exercise. Her LDL value is much improved, but her glucose value is 140.*

**What new diagnosis might she have?**

Diabetes mellitus

**Which type?**

Type 2

**How does type 2 DM present?**

Often in obese patients after the age of 40 with gradual onset of symptoms (polyuria, polyphagia, polydipsia, and weight loss) or with an abnormal lab test

**What's the basic mechanism causing the disease?**

Defects in insulin receptors

**What are some common secondary causes of DM?**

Medications (steroids, thiazide diuretics, etc.) and pancreatic insufficiency

**Which type of DM has a stronger genetic predisposition?**

Type 2 greater than type 1 owing to 90% concordance rate in monozygotic twins

**How is the diagnosis made in**
 **Asymptomatic patients?**

Either by a fasting plasma glucose greater than 126 mg/dL on two separate occasions or by a positive 2-hour oral glucose tolerance test (2 values at 2 hours exceed 200 mg/dL)

 **Symptomatic patients?**

Presence of symptoms (weight loss, polyuria, etc.) with a random plasma glucose greater than 200 mg/dL

**What is the initial treatment?**

Diabetic diet (60% carbohydrates, 15% protein, and 25% fat not exceeding 35 kcal/kg/day) and physical activity to attain ideal body weight

**How is the DM monitored?**

Numerous daily capillary blood glucose measurements

**What are the recommended fasting, preprandial, and postprandial glucose levels?**

Fasting and preprandial between 70 and 120 mg/dL and postprandial less than 160 mg/dL

| | |
|---|---|
| **What lab test is used to assess glycemic control over the last 4 weeks?** | Glycosylated hemoglobin $A_1C$ |
| **What is the next therapy in type 2 DM?** | Oral hypoglycemic agents such as metformin (glucophage) and acarbose (precose) followed by insulin if needed |
| **What additional appointments should be made for recently diagnosed diabetics?** | Dietary consult, yearly eye and foot exams |

## CASE 3

*A 38-year-old female with history of chronic obstructive pulmonary disease (COPD), hypertension, and type 1 diabetes with retinopathy and renal insufficiency secondary to poor compliance with her insulin regimen is brought to the ER by her husband saying that she was complaining of symptoms similar to when her diabetes was diagnosed, but also had some nausea and vomiting and vague abdominal pain. Within the last few hours she has begun to breath rapidly with a fruity smell to her breath and seems to be a bit confused.*

| | |
|---|---|
| **What is most likely causing this patient's symptoms?** | Diabetic ketoacidosis (DKA) |
| **What's in the differential diagnosis when considering DKA?** | Salicylate poisoning (aspirin overdose), metabolic acidosis from methyl alcohol, ethylene glycol ingestion, uremic acidosis, alcoholic ketoacidosis |
| **How does DKA often present?** | Polyuria, polydipsia, unexplained weight loss, vomiting, and vague abdominal pain followed by hyperventilation (Kussmaul sign), shock, and coma if untreated |
| **Why does DKA occur?** | Extremely low levels of insulin lead to hyperglycemia, hyperglucagonemia, increased stress hormones, and ketoacid production by the liver |

| | |
|---|---|
| **Is it more common in type 1 or type 2 diabetes?** | Type 1 |
| **Why is it less common in type 2 diabetics?** | They usually make enough insulin to prevent DKA from developing. |
| **What is the most likely cause in this patient?** | Noncompliance with her insulin regimen |
| **What were the clues to non-compliance in the patient?** | Patient has developed at least two chronic complications from her underlying disease which suggests poor disease control and possible noncompliance with taking her insulin |
| **What other triggers to DKA must be considered?** | Stress (often infection), myocardial infarction (MI), or cerebral vascular accident (CVA) |
| **What might the PE reveal in DKA patients?** | Altered mental status, fruity breath odor (from acetone), signs of dehydration (tachycardia, dry mucous membranes, poor skin turgor), tachypnea (Kussmaul respiration), evidence of infection (e.g., diabetic ulcer, pneumonia, pyelonephritis) |
| **What should you order?**<br>   **Labs** | STAT acucheck, serum electrolytes, serum ketones, arterial blood gas, CBC, and blood cultures (if infection suspected) |
|    **Tests/imaging** | EKG to evaluate possible MI or hyperkalemia, and CXR if infection is suspected |
| **How is it diagnosed?** | Hyperglycemia, hyperketonemia, and metabolic acidosis with an elevated anion gap |
| **What is the treatment?** | Admit for IV fluids and insulin, K supplementation as needed |

## CASE 4

*A 55-year-old male with history of gastroesophageal reflux disease (GERD), esophagitis, hypertension, and diabetes is admitted to the hospital for confusion and an acucheck of 850 without an anion gap.*

**What's his most likely diagnosis?**

Nonketotic hyperosmolar coma

**Does this occur in type 1 or type 2 diabetics?**

Type 2

**How does it present?**

Polyuria, polydipsia, lethargic, obtunded or coma with severe hyperglycemia (600 to 2000 mg/100 mL) dehydration

**How is it distinguished from DKA?**

Absence of ketoacidosis (no fruity breath or hyperventilation)

**Why does ketoacidosis not occur?**

Type 2 diabetics make enough insulin to prevent lipolysis and ketoacid production.

**What causes the symptoms in nonketotic hyperosmolar coma?**

Hyperglycemia, dehydration, and hyperosmolality

**What can precipitate it?**

Stress, stroke, excessive carbohydrate intake, or infection

**What might be found on physical exam?**

Altered mental status, signs of dehydration (tachycardia, dry mucous membranes, poor skin turgor), evidence of infection (e.g., diabetic ulcer, pneumonia, pyelonephritis), or stroke

**What should you order?**
  **Labs**

STAT acucheck, serum electrolytes, serum ketones, arterial blood gas, CBC, and blood cultures (if infection suspected)

  **Tests/imaging**

EKG to evaluate possible MI or hyperkalemia, and CXR if infection is suspected

| | |
|---|---|
| **How is it diagnosed?** | Hyperglycemia without elevated serum ketones or anion gap |
| **What is the treatment?** | IVF and parenteral insulin with rigorous blood glucose monitoring |
| **What electrolyte abnormality are patients at risk for with insulin?** | Hypokalemia |
| **What is the treatment?** | Potassium supplementation |

## DISEASES OF THE THYROID AND PARATHYROID GLAND

### CASE 5

*A 72-year-old male with history of psoriasis, gout, and dementia presents to the clinic for routine checkup and complains of intermittent anxiety, sweating, fatigue, headache, and mild confusion. The symptoms occur usually in the morning and after he takes his medications, which include insulin, hydrochlorathizide, aspirin, and lipitor. The symptoms lessen after eating breakfast.*

| | |
|---|---|
| **What are the patients symptoms consistent with?** | Hypoglycemia |
| **What are the symptoms and signs of** | |
| **Mild hypoglycemia?** | Anxiety, diaphoresis, tachycardia, lethargy, confusion, and headache |
| **Severe hypoglycemia?** | Mild symptoms followed by seizure, stupor, coma, or focal neurologic findings |
| **How is the diagnosis of hypoglycemia made?** | Hypoglycemic symptoms with a low glucose level that are relieved with treatment |
| **What's the differential diagnosis for hypoglycemia?** | Insulinoma, insulin use, sulfonylurea use, postgastrectomy patients |

| | |
|---|---|
| **Which is most likely in this patient?** | Insulin use |
| **What labs are ordered when the cause is unclear?** | Plasma insulin level, insulin antibodies, plasma/urine sulfonylurea levels, C-peptide |
| **What's the diagnosis with** | |
|    **High plasma insulin level with insulin antibodies?** | Exogenous insulin use |
|    **Plasma or urine sulfo-nylurea levels positive?** | Oral sulfonylurea use |
|    **Elevated C-peptide?** | Insulinoma |
| **What is the treatment for** | |
|    **Mild hypoglycemia?** | Oral carbohydrates (fruit, fruit juice, crackers, etc.) |
|    **Severe hypoglycemia?** | IV $D_{50}$ solution or SC/IM glucagon if IV access is not available |
|    **Diabetic and drug-related cause?** | Adjust drug therapy, diet, and physical activity |
|    **Insulinoma?** | Pancreatic spiral CT, arteriography, or ultrasonography (transabdominal and endoscopic) to localize lesion followed by surgical referral |

## CASE 6

*A 62-year-old woman with history of diabetes, bipolar disorder controlled with lithium, COPD secondary to lung cancer, atrial fibrillation controlled with amiodarone, esophageal cancer s/p chemotherapy and radiation presents to clinic with complaints of fatigue, weight gain, and slow bowels. You notice she is wearing a fall coat in the summer. She says it helps her keep warm.*

| | |
|---|---|
| **What underlying disease do you suspect?** | Hypothyroidism |

**How does it present?**

Often nonspecific symptoms including cold intolerance, fatigue, weight gain, paresthesias (hand and feet), constipation, muscle weakness, muscle cramps, arthralgias, and hoarseness

**What is it?**

A hypometabolic condition that results from a decrease in thyroid hormone at the cellular level

**What risk factors does she have?**

History of prior neck radiation and surgery, drugs (amiodarone and lithium can cause hypothyroidism)

**What other risk factors may be presented to you?**

Other drugs (iodine, $\alpha$-interferon and interleukin-2), Hashimoto thyroiditis, and pituitary disease

**What is a clue that a patient may have received iodine?**

Recent radiographic imaging using contrast dye (some contain iodine)

**What physical exam findings support hypothyroidism?**

Bradycardia, hypothermia, periorbital edema, dry skin, nonpitting edema, and decreased tendon reflexes (prolonged relaxation)

**What's the best single screening test for hypothyroidism?**

Thyroid-stimulating hormone (TSH)

**What result do you expect?**

High plasma TSH

**What additional test confirms primary hypothyroidism?**

Decreased free T4 or FTI (free thyroxine index)

**How is secondary hypothyroidism (pituitary disease) diagnosed?**

Normal TSH with a decreased T4 index

**What is the treatment?**

Thyroxine (T4; Synthroid, Levothroid, Levoxyl), start at 50–100 µg/day unless elderly or CAD and then start with 25 µg/day and slowly taper up until TSH level is normalized

| | |
|---|---|
| **What is a possible complication of hypothyroidism?** | Myxedema crisis |
| **What can cause it?** | Infection (common), trauma, and cold exposure |
| **How does it present?** | Hypothermia, hyporeflexia, bradycardia, hypotension, hyponatremia, and hypoventilation |
| **What is the treatment?** | IV thyroxine |
| **What additional treatment is suggested in secondary hypothyroidism?** | Hydrocortisone (decreases risk of concomitant adrenal insufficiency) |

## CASE 7

*A 41-year-old previously healthy female comes to your office with her husband complaining of feeling nervous and anxious along with a periodic heart pounding in her chest, difficulty sleeping, and feeling hot all the time. Her husband adds additional concerns that her eyes are bulging out and she has non-pitting leg swelling over her shins.*

| | |
|---|---|
| **What do you think she has?** | Hyperthyroidism |
| **What is it?** | A disease characterized by excess free-thyroid hormone in the body due to a hyperfunctioning thyroid gland |
| **What are some common symptoms?** | Palpitations (heart pounding), anxiety, nervousness, insomnia, heat intolerance, increased sweating, weight loss, hair loss, and frequent bowel movements |
| **What's the differential diagnosis for hyperthyroidism?** | Graves disease, excess medication, toxic nodular goiter, thyroiditis, and cancer (papillary type most common in the thyroid gland, as well as TSH-secreting pituitary tumors) |
| **What is the most common cause?** | Graves disease (γ-immunoglobins bind to TSH receptors) |

| | |
|---|---|
| **Who is at increased risk of Graves disease?** | Middle-aged women |
| **What clues in the presentation help you narrow your differential diagnosis?** | Eyes bulging (exopthalamus) and nonpitting leg swelling (pretibial myxedema) |
| **How so?** | These physical exam signs are specific to Graves disease. |
| **What additional signs may be apparent on physical exam?** | Goiter, tachycardia, fine tremor, stare, eyelid lag, atrial fibrillation, warm skin, and brisk tendon reflexes |
| **What labs should you order?** | TSH, Free T4 or T4 index |
| **What's diagnostic of hyperthyroidism?** | Low TSH (less than 0.1 μU/mL) and high T4 or T4 index |
| **What diagnostic tests can be ordered if cancer is suspected?** | Fine needle aspiration and thyroid scans |
| **What is the pharmacologic therapy for hyperthyroidism?** | Long-term therapy with the antithyroid drugs methimazole and propylthiouracil (PTU) |
| **What is their mechanism of action?** | While both inhibit thyroid hormone synthesis, PTU also inhibits conversion of T4 to T3. |
| **What nuclear medicine therapy is available?** | One or two doses of radioactive iodine (RAI) to impair thyroid hormone synthesis over the next several months |
| **What surgical treatment is available when medical therapy fails or patient refuses RAI therapy?** | Subtotal thyroidectomy |
| **What is the dreaded complication of Graves disease?** | Thyroid storm (often triggered by stress or infection), a medical emergency |
| **How does thyroid storm present?** | Fever, tachycardia, weakness, delirium, and shock |

| **What is the treatment?** | IV fluids, steroids, PTU, potassium iodide, and a β-blocker |

## CASE 8

*A 71-year-old female is brought to the doctor by her son after he noticed a letter sent to his mother regarding an endocrine health fair she attended where various screening tests were performed for free in an effort to offer enrollment to patients in experimental studies. The letter informed her she should see her doctor due to an elevated calcium and parathyroid hormone (PTH). She informs you she feels fine and saw no reason to bother you with this. She only went to the health fair to have her arthritic knees evaluated.*

| **What's her most likely diagnosis?** | Primary hyperparathyroidism |
| **Is her presentation consistent with the diagnosis?** | Yes, most often patients are asymptomatic middle-aged or elderly women with an abnormal screening test, but some present with "painful bones, renal stones, abdominal groans, and psychic overtones" if PTH is >13 mg/dL. |
| **What hormone causes primary hyperparathyroidism?** | Increased PTH secretion resulting in hypercalcemia |
| **What's the most common cause?** | Parathyroid adenoma |
| **What are less common causes?** | Parathyroid hyperplasia or carcinoma |
| **What should be done first?** | Confirm the diagnosis |
| **What labs should be ordered?** | Serum PTH, calcium, and phosphorus at a minimum |
| **What is the diagnosis made?** | Hypercalcemia (on at least 2 occasions), hypophosphatemia, and elevated PTH |
| **What additional laboratory finding may be found?** | Elevated alkaline phosphatase (in patients with significant bone disease) and hypercalciuria |

| | |
|---|---|
| **What radiographic imaging should you order?** | Neck ultrasound and CT to look for parathyroid adenomas |
| **What is the treatment if serum calcium rises above 13 to 15 mg/dL or patient is symptomatic?** | IVF and furosemide, parenteral salmon calcitonin, pamidronate (bisphosphonate with antiresorbtive properties), mithramycin (inhibits bone resorption), and phosphate |
| **What is the definitive treatment for patients with serum calcium levels above 11 mg/dL?** | Parathyroidectomy |

## CASE 9

*A 68-year-old female with history of diabetes, gout, and thyroid cancer s/p partial thyroidectomy presents with slow onset of tingling of her lips and fingers 3 weeks after surgery. Her husband thinks it's related to her uncontrolled diabetes.*

| | |
|---|---|
| **What do you think?** | More likely to be hypoparathyroidism secondary to accidental removal of parathyroid glands during thyroid surgery causing hypocalcemia |
| **What other conditions can cause hypocalcemia?** | Renal insufficiency, hypoalbuminemia, vitamin D deficiency, hypomagnesemia, pancreatitis, hyperphosphatemia, pseudohypoparathyroidism, autosomal recessive causing end-organ resistance to PTH, sepsis, large blood transfusion (from EDTA in blood) |
| **Describe the following signs on physical exam that suggest hypocalcemia.** | |
| Chvostek sign | Tapping cheek results in facial twitch |
| Trousseau sign | Carpal spasm occurs just minutes after blood pressure cuff is inflated |

| | |
|---|---|
| **What basic labs should you order?** | Chem 8, phosphorus, albumin, and PTH |
| **What result is diagnostic of hypoparathyroidism?** | Low PTH and Ca with high phosphorus |
| **What's the treatment?** | Ca and vitamin D supplementation |

## MISCELLANEOUS DISORDERS

### CASE 10

*A 13-year-old previously healthy Caucasian boy presents to your clinic with history of progressive weakness and weight loss. His mother thinks it's related to his decreased appetite. You notice the child appears quite tan and is orthostatic on vital signs.*

| | |
|---|---|
| **What do you suspect?** | Primary adrenocortical insufficiency |
| **What's the etiology?** | Insufficient steroid output from the adrenal cortex due to a disease of the adrenal glands (primary failure) or to disorders of the pituitary or hypothalamus (secondary failure) |
| **How does it commonly present?** | Anorexia, nausea, vomiting, weakness, weight loss, fatigue |
| **What clues in the presentation helped narrow your differential diagnosis and specify primary adrenal failure as the most likely cause?** | Hyperpigmentation (due to excess ACTH) and orthostasis indicating volume depletion (due to hyponatremia secondary to aldosterone deficiency) |
| **Why does hyperpigmentation occur in primary disease?** | Adrenocorticotropic hormone (ACTH) and melanocyte-stimulating hormone (MSH) are derived from the same precursor, so when ACTH production goes up, so does MSH, which leads to hyperpigmented skin |

**What additional features may only occur in primary adrenal failure?**

Hypoglycemia and hyperkalemia

**What presentation in the ER should significantly increase your suspicion of primary adrenocortical insufficiency?**

A hypotensive orthostatic patient with hyperpigmentation who fails to respond to fluids and has hyponatremia, hyperkalemia, or hypoglycemia of unknown etiology

**What's the differential diagnosis for causes of**

**Primary adrenal failure?**

Autoimmune destruction (Addison disease most common), infection (HIV, fungal, tuberculosis), hemorrhagic adrenal infarction (anticoagulant therapy), metastasis

**Secondary adrenal failure?**

Glucocorticoid therapy and pituitary failure due to a disease process or to surgery (two most common causes)

**Who is at increased risk of secondary causes of adrenocortical insufficiency?**

AIDS patients (disseminated infection or ketoconazole treatment) or steroid-dependent patients with abrupt withdrawal of their exogenous steroids

**What initial labs should you order?**

Chem 8, CBC, 24-hour urinary cortisol, 17-OHCS, 17-KS, and ACTH

**What findings support the diagnosis of adrenal insufficiency on**

**Chem 8?**

Increased $K^+$, decreased $Na^+$ and $Cl^-$, decreased glucose, increased BUN:creatinine ratio (pre-renal azotemia)

**CBC?**

Mild normocytic, normochromic anemia

**24-hour urinary cortisol, 17-OHCS, and 17-KS?**

Decreased

**ACTH?**

Increased in primary adrenocortical insufficiency

| | |
|---|---|
| **How is it diagnosed?** | Inadequate response to cortrosyn (ACTH) stimulation test (cortisol level does not increase after administration of ACTH) |
| **What lab results distinguish primary and secondary causes?** | Primary causes have elevated ACTH and low aldosterone; secondary causes have low ACTH and normal aldosterone |
| **What is the treatment?** | Hydrocortisone |
| **What additional treatment is required if hypoaldosteronism exists (primary disease)?** | A mineralocorticoid-like fludrocortisone (Florinef) |

## CASE 11

*A 35-year-old female comes to your clinic complaining of fatigue, weakness, and feeling depressed over the last few months. She feels depressed over her appearance. On physical exam you appreciate truncal obesity, rounded face, thin, faint facial hair, acne, a few abdominal striae, and bruises on her arms and legs.*

| | |
|---|---|
| **What do these findings suggest?** | Cushing syndrome |
| **What is Cushing syndrome?** | A syndrome characterized primarily by effects of excess cortisol, although excess mineralocorticoids and androgenic steroids may also be present |
| **What causes it?** | Administration of exogenous glucocorticoids (most common) or by excess production of cortisol by the adrenal cortex |
| **What lung disease is associated with Cushing syndrome?** | Oat-cell lung cancer can produce ACTH, which stimulates the adrenal cortex to produce excess cortisol |
| **What is Cushing disease?** | Excess cortisol production from the adrenal cortex caused by increased ACTH secreted by the pituitary, often from a pituitary microadenoma |

| | |
|---|---|
| **What is the best screening test for Cushing syndrome?** | A 24-hour urine free-cortisol level (elevated in Cushing syndrome) |
| **What was the test used before 24-hour urine free-cortisol testing became common practice?** | 1–2 mg overnight dexamethasone suppression test |
| **If the screening test (24-hour urine free-cortisol) is positive, what test is ordered next?** | Serum ACTH level |
| **Why?** | You're trying to determine if the elevated cortisol level is ACTH dependent (Cushing disease) or independent (ACTH from lung cancer, for example) |

**How do you interpret the following results?**

| | |
|---|---|
| **Normal 24-hour urine cortisol and normal ACTH** | Not Cushing syndrome |
| **High 24-hour urine cortisol and normal or high ACTH** | ACTH-dependent Cushing syndrome |
| **High cortisol with suppressed ACTH** | ACTH-independent Cushing syndrome |
| **What additional test is needed in the ACTH-dependent Cushing group?** | High-dose dexamethasone test |
| **What are you trying to determine?** | If the ACTH is produced by the pituitary (Cushing disease) or an ectopic source (e.g., lung cancer) |
| **What lab values indicate a positive high-dose dexamethasone test?** | Decreased levels of urinary cortisol or 17-hydroxycorticosteroids following administration of high-dose dexamethasone |

**What's your diagnosis with a positive result?**     Cushing disease

**What imaging is ordered for Cushing disease?**     CT or MRI of pituitary

**ACTH-dependent Cushing syndrome with negative dexamethasone suppression test?**     CT or MRI of chest (looking for ectopic ACTH-producing tumors)

**ACTH-independent Cushing syndrome?**     Adrenal CT or MRI

**What's the definitive treatment in all conditions?**     Surgery

**What's the type of surgery in Cushing disease?**     Transsphenoidal microadenectomy

**What treatment is available for nonsurgical Cushing disease patients?**     Pituitary irradiation

## CASE 12

*You've been signed out a 36-year-old female with history of torn right knee ACL s/p surgery years ago who presents to the ER today with her husband complaining of worsening headache over the last few months. At first it was relieved with over-the-counter (OTC) ibuprofen and Tylenol, but over the last few weeks it has become progressively worse and the OTC meds are not helping. She came to the ER today because she developed temporary visual loss and double vision that lasted for 1 hour earlier in the morning. A CT of the head is suggestive of a pituitary or sellar mass lesion.*

**What can cause this finding?**     Benign pituitary adenoma, infiltrative disease, autoimmune phenomena, hypothalamic

**Which hormones are usually affected by functioning pituitary tumors?**     ACTH, growth hormone (GH), and prolactin (PRL, most common)

| | |
|---|---|
| **Which hormones are rarely affected?** | TSH, follicle-stimulating hormone, and luteinizing hormone |
| **Other than calling neurosurgery to review the film, what additional findings would support the CT findings?** | Elevated prolactin (hyperprolactinemia), GH (acromegaly), or ACTH (Cushing syndrome) excess |
| **How would hyperprolactinemia commonly present?** | Galactorrhea and amenorrhea in women (impotence and loss of libido in men) |
| **How does excess GH present?** | Acromegaly in adults resulting in large jaw, forehead, and hands (gigantism in children) |
| **How does excess ACTH present?** | Cushing syndrome (see Cushing disease case) |
| **What lab results suggest the diagnosis?** | Abnormal level of GH, PRL, or ACTH |
| **What lab test strongly suggests the diagnosis in GH-producing tumors?** | Glucose challenge test |
| **What additional diagnostic imaging test will the neurosurgeon recommend?** | MRI (preferred over CT) |
| **What medical therapy may be used to control small PRL-secreting adenomas?** | Bromocriptine |
| **When is transsphenoidal surgery with or without radiation warranted?** | In cases of hormone excess or neurologic symptoms |
| **What additional therapy may be required in hypopitarianism ?** | Hormone replacement |

## CASE 13

*You're called by the neurosurgery team for a consult on a 24-year-old male who was hospitalized 5 days ago after a severe motor vehicle collision resulting in several bone fractures, including a basilar skull fracture. The consult is for significant imbalance in body fluid input and output. For days he has been making large quantities of dilute urine which has required up to 6 L of saline to keep up with losses.*

| | |
|---|---|
| **What is your differential diagnosis?** | Diabetes insipidus, diabetes mellitus, polydipsia, osmotic diuresis (glucose, mannitol, urea) |
| **Which diagnosis do you suspect?** | Diabetes insipidus (DI) |
| **Why?** | Large quantity of dilute urine after sustaining significant head trauma (basilar skull fracture) is a risk factor for DI |
| **Name some other risk factors for DI.** | Neurosurgical procedures, brain tumors, and drugs (ethanol, phenytoin, or lithium) |
| **Other than polyuria, what do you expect the patient to complain of with DI?** | Excessive thirst |
| **What are the two types of DI?** | Neurogenic and nephrogenic |
| **What causes neurogenic DI?** | Insufficient release of vasopressin by the pituitary |
| **What causes nephrogenic DI?** | Distal nephron does not respond to vasopressin |
| **Which is more likely in this patient?** | Neurogenic DI |
| **What do you expect to find on physical exam?** | Dehydration, hypovolemia with large quantity of urine output recorded by the nurses |

| | |
|---|---|
| **How is the diagnosis of DI made?** | Dilute urine and increased serum osmolality |
| **What test is ordered to distinguish between central and nephrogenic DI?** | Water deprivation test |
| **What is the treatment for symptomatic neurogenic DI?** | The intranasal vasopressin analog desamino-8-D-arginine vasopression (DDAVP, Desmopressin) |
| **What is the treatment for nephrogenic DI?** | Hydration and thiazide diuretics |

## CASE 14

*A 63-year-old male with history of arthritis, carpal tunnel, COPD secondary to smoking, and benign prostatic hypertrophy (BPH) presents to the hospital after falling off his bike. For months, as part of an exercise program, he has biked 5–10 miles daily down a straight gravel path, but stopped 5 days ago as a result of significant muscle weakness and cramping. In the ER he received a battery of lab tests and a simple CXR. The chemistry panel revealed hyponatremia and the CXR had RML lesion consistent with underlying lung cancer.*

| | |
|---|---|
| **What's the most likely diagnosis?** | Syndrome of inappropriate antidiuretic hormone secretion (SIADH) secondary to underlying lung cancer |
| **How can SIADH present?** | With symptoms of hyponatremia, such as lethargy, muscle cramps, confusion, headache, focal neurologic findings, convulsions, and coma |
| **What's his main risk factor?** | Smoking |
| **Which type of lung cancer is this associated with?** | Oat-cell carcinoma of the lung |
| **What are some other risk factors for SIADH?** | Pulmonary diseases (e.g., pneumonia, tuberculosis), stroke, head lesion (tumor, trauma, infection), and drugs (e.g., chlorpropamide, carbamazepine, and diuretics) |

| | |
|---|---|
| **What labs should you order?** | Chem 8, serum and urinary and serum osmolarity |
| **What are the associated lab findings?** | Hyponatremia with a urinary osmolarity greater than serum osmolarity |
| **How is the diagnosis made?** | With the associated lab findings after all other causes have been ruled out (e.g., diuretics, dehydration, anterior pituitary, renal, adrenal, and thyroid disease) |
| **What is the initial treatment?** | Correct underlying cause (most likely lung cancer in this case) and fluid restriction |

## CASE 15

*A 55-year-old Asian female with history of emphysema secondary to smoking, RA in remission on methotrexate and prednisone for years presents to the clinic after being discharged from the ER with a wrist fracture after falling in her kitchen.*

| | |
|---|---|
| **What underlying disease does she most likely have that put her at risk of the wrist fracture?** | Osteoporosis |
| **What risk factors does she have?** | Age, postmenopausal, smoker, chronic steroid use, Asian (Hispanics also at increased risk) |
| **What are some secondary causes of osteoporosis?** | Hyperthyroidism, hyperparathyroidism, osteomalacia, multiple myeloma, and medications (glucocorticoids most common, as well as T4 overreplacement) |
| **How do most cases present?** | Usually asymptomatic until fracture occurs |
| **Which fractures are most common?** | Vertebral, wrist (Colles fracture), and hip fractures |

**What test should you order to diagnose osteoporosis?**

Dual-energy x-ray absorptiometry (DXA) bone scan to measure bone mineral density

**What are the 2 scores reported in DXA scans?**

T and Z score

**What are they?**
  **T score**

Number of standard deviations from the mean for young, normal controls

  **Z score**

Number of standard deviations from the mean for an age- and sex-matched control group

**How is osteoporosis diagnosed?**

T score more than 2 standard deviations below the mean

**What's the therapy?**

Calcium and vitamin D supplements, bisphosphonate treatment (alendronate and resedronate), weight-bearing exercise, stop smoking, discontinue offending medications, and consider hormone replacement therapy (not first-line therapy) if fails to improve on standard therapy

**What test should be ordered to gauge response to therapy?**

DXA scan

**When?**

1 year after therapy initiated

# 6 Hematology and Oncology

## MALIGNANT NEOPLASMS

*A 58-year-old male with history of chronic obstructive pulmonary disease (COPD), hypertension (HTN), and lung cancer s/p resection, radiation, and chemotherapy years ago presents with profound fatigue, generalized weakness, dyspnea on exertion, fever, petechiae, and easy bruising.*

| | |
|---|---|
| **What's your differential diagnosis?** | Lung cancer recurrence with metastasis, anemia, acute leukemia |
| **Which is most likely?** | Acute leukemia |
| **Why?** | Because low levels of WBC, Hg, and PLT can explain all his symptoms |

**What symptoms may occur with the following in acute leukemia?**

| | |
|---|---|
| **Leukopenia** | Fever, infection, and sepsis |
| **Anemia** | Fatigue, pallor, and dyspnea |
| **Thrombocytopenia** | Purpura, bleeding, petechiae |
| **What risk factors does the patient have for acute leukemia?** | Radiation and chemotherapy exposure |
| **What other risk factors should be remembered?** | Down syndrome and benzene |
| **If acute leukemia is diagnosed, which type does he most likely have?** | Acute myelogenous leukemia (AML) |
| **Why?** | It is more common in the elderly, whereas ALL (acute lymphoblastic leukemia) is more common in children. |

**What findings on physical exam would support the diagnosis of acute leukemia?**

Splenomegaly, hepatometomegaly, lymphadenopathy, and bone tenderness

**Do all these need to be present?**

No

**What tests should you order?**

CBC, LDH, peripheral blood smear; pan culture (blood and urine) and CXR due to fever and type and cross for possible transfusion

**What results will support the diagnosis of acute leukemia in the**
    **CBC?**

Pancytopenia (low WBC, Hg, PLT) supporting bone marrow pathology

    **LDH?**

Elevated (indicative of cell death in leukemia)

**The history, physical exam, and basic lab tests suggest acute leukemia. What will clinch the diagnosis?**

Blasts in the peripheral blood smear or in bone marrow aspirate (presence of greater than 30% in the bone marrow)

**AML is confirmed. What caused it?**

A malignant neoplasm of the blood-forming organs characterized by diffuse replacement of bone marrow with proliferating leukocyte precursors resulting in abnormal numbers and forms or immature white cells in circulation

**What is the supportive therapy for**
    **Septic or a low neutrophil count?**

Broad-spectrum antibiotics

    **Active bleeding or platelet count <20,000/µL?**

Platelet transfusion

    **Severe anemia?**

RBC transfusion

| | |
|---|---|
| **What is the definitive therapy?** | Chemotherapy and bone marrow transplant |

## CASE 2

*A 47-year-old male with history of benign prostatic hypertrophy (BPH), HTN, and degenerative joint disease (DJD) presents to the office for a yearly physical, and basic lab review done prior to the visit revealed a WBC count of 105,000. The patient says he feels fine and has not noticed any limitations in his usual routine.*

| | |
|---|---|
| **What are you concerned about?** | Leukemia |
| **What type?** | Chronic myelogenous leukemia (CML) |
| **Why?** | Elevated WBC of greater than 100,000 is highly suspicious for CML; roughly 40% of patients are asymptomatic on presentation and the median age at presentation is 45. |
| **What causes CML?** | A malignant myeloproliferation of the hematopoietic stem cells |
| **As CML progresses, what type of leukemias are patients at risk of developing?** | AML and ALL |
| **What finding on physical exam would support the diagnosis of CML?** | Splenomegaly |
| **Name the three phases of CML.** | Chronic, accelerated, and blast |
| **Which stage is this patient in?** | Chronic |
| **Name common symptoms that CML patients may present with.** | Anemia (pallor, fatigue, and dyspnea on exertion), weight loss, low-grade fevers, night sweats, mild upper left quadrant discomfort (associated splenomegaly) |

| | |
|---|---|
| **You know the WBC is elevated. What additional serologic tests should you order now to support your diagnosis?** | Leukocyte alkaline phosphatase, LDH |
| **What result do you expect for leukocyte alkaline phosphatase?** | Decreased |
| **LDH?** | Increased |
| **What is the significance of low leukocyte alkaline phosphatase?** | Distinguishes CML from other myeloproliferative disorders |
| **What additional CBC abnormalities may be found?** | Normochromic-normocytic anemia (mild) and thrombocytosis |
| **Your labs and physical exam support the diagnosis of CML. What must be done to confirm the diagnosis?** | (1) Bone marrow biopsy (2) Cytologic and chromosomal analysis |
| **What findings are required on Bone marrow biopsy?** | Hypercellular bone marrow with granulocyte hyperplasia, increased ratio of myeloid cells to erythroid cells, increased megakaryocytes with few blasts and promyelocytes |
| **Cytologic and chromosomal analysis?** | The Philadelphia chromosome (9:22 chromosomal translocation) or its products, the BCR/ABL fusion mRNA, and the Bcr/Abl protein |
| **Chronic phase of CML is diagnosed. What's your treatment plan?** | Palliative therapy with chemotherapy (hydroxyurea, decreases leukocytosis and thromocytosis) and α-interferon (decreases number of cells carrying Philadelphia chromosome) or combination of interferon and cytosine arabinoside |

| | |
|---|---|
| **What is the natural progression of CML?** | Chronic phase to accelerated and blast phase |
| **What treatment may prevent disease progression?** | Bone marrow transplant |
| **What symptoms and signs indicate they are likely progressing into the blast phase?** | Increased chronic phase symptoms with lymphadenopathy, bone pain, marked anemia, thrombocytopenia (easy bruising), and predominance of blasts |
| **What are blast phase patients at risk for?** | Infection and bleeding due to bone marrow failure (most often causes of death) |
| **What treatments are available for the accelerated and blast phases?** | Intensive chemotherapy, leukopheresis, and bone marrow transplant; most treatments fail |

## CASE 3

*A 64-year-old male with history of hypertension s/p successful treatment for upper respiratory tract infection (URTI) is noted to have elevated WBC of 5500 with predominance of lymphocytes.*

| | |
|---|---|
| **What differential diagnosis are you considering?** | Chronic lymphocytic leukemia (CLL), hairy cell leukemia, and Waldenström macroglobulinemia |
| **Which diagnosis do you suspect?** | CLL |
| **Why?** | Median age at presentation is 65 (patient is 64) and patients often present asymptomatic with elevated lymphocytes |
| **What causes CLL?** | Monoclonal expansion of immunoincompetent B lymphocytes (rarely T lymphocytes) into the peripheral blood, bone marrow, spleen, and lymph nodes |
| **What's your diagnostic workup for CLL?** | CBC with smear and differential, cell marker studies |

**Describe the diagnostic findings by**

    **CBC with differential and smear**

Lymphocyte count greater than 5000/μL

    **Peripheral smear**

Monoclonal proliferation of lymphocytes

    **Cell markers**

Positive B-cell antigens CD19 and CD20 along with the T-cell antigen CD5

**The diagnosis of CLL is confirmed by the above studies. Will you recommend treatment now?**

No

**Why?**

Treatment indications are not met.

**What are they?**

Neutropenia, recurrent infection, anemia, thrombocytopenia, constitutional symptoms, massive splenomegaly, and massive lymphadenopathy causing discomfort

**Why are CLL patents prone to infections?**

Decreased levels of immunoglobulins and impaired cellular immunity

**What's your management plan for this patient with early-stage CLL?**

Observation for signs or symptoms of disease progression with consideration for IV immunoglobins if hypogammaglobulinemia is present to decrease risk of infection

**What symptoms may the patient develop as the disease progresses?**

Symptoms of anemia (fatigue, pallor, dyspnea on exertion), thrombocytopenia (easy bruising and gingival bleeding), fever, night sweats, weight loss, splenomegaly, and lymphadenopathy

**What therapy will you recommend once he develops signs and symptoms of advanced-stage CLL?**

Chemotherapy with consideration for allogeneic stem cell transplantation

**What is the median survival after diagnosis?**

6 years

## CASE 4

*A 28-year-old previously healthy female is referred to you from a family practitioner in a rural setting for further workup of a painless lump around her bra strap above the collar bone. She denies any associated symptoms of URTI, fever, chills, or constitutional symptoms. On exam you find 2 nontender supraclavicular nodes, a Band-Aid where the referring physician biopsed one of the superficial nodes, and mild hepatosplenomegaly.*

| | |
|---|---|
| **What's your differential diagnosis?** | Infected furuncle, throat infection, dental abscess, cat-scratch fever, lymphoma (Hodgkin lymphoma and non-Hodgkin lymphoma), AIDS/HIV infection |
| **Which do you suspect?** | Lymphoma |
| **Why?** | It often presents with isolated painless swelling of a lymph node in the neck, axilla, or groin, which then spreads to adjacent groups of lymph nodes; hepatosplenomegaly may be found. No evidence on physical exam of other underlying infection was found. |
| **What basic labs should be included in your workup?** | CBC, Chem 8, liver function tests, ESR, and HIV (if risk factors are present; not in this patient) |
| **Your nurse passes you the pathology report from the biopsy taken last week and it says Reed-Sternberg cells were found. What is this pathognomonic for?** | Hodgkin disease (non-Hodgkin disease lacks Reed-Sternberg cells) |
| **What causes Hodgkin disease?** | Malignancy of the lymphatic system secondary to monoclonal proliferation of B cells |
| **Does this patient have type A or B (A or B symptoms)?** | Type A (asymptomatic) due to lack of constitutional symptoms; Type B has B symptoms |

| | |
|---|---|
| **Name the common B symptoms.** | Fever, chills, night sweats, and weight loss |
| **What do B symptoms suggest?** | Advanced disease |
| **Is any further testing required to make the diagnosis?** | No. Lymph node biopsy (already done) is the gold standard diagnostic test. |
| **What additional tests are required to stage her disease?** | CT scan, gallium or PET scan, bilateral bone marrow biopsy, and aspiration |
| **Imaging states a region of lymphadenopathy is limited to one side of the diaphragm. What stage does she have?** | Stage I |
| **Define the other stages.** | |
| **Stage II** | Two lymph node regions on one side of diaphragm |
| **Stage III** | Lymph node regions on both sides of diaphragm |
| **Stage IV** | Disseminated disease with bone marrow or liver involvement |
| **What's the treatment for your patient with stage I disease?** | Local radiation |
| **What's the treatment for stage** | |
| **IIA?** | Radiation |
| **IIB?** | Radiation and chemotherapy |
| **III and IV?** | Chemotherapy |

## CASE 5

*A 65-year-old African American male with history of BPH presents with decreased stream strength, sensation of incomplete voiding, blood in urine, unintentional weight loss, and mid-back pain.*

| | |
|---|---|
| **What's the differential diagnosis?** | Urinary tract infection (UTI), BPH, prostatitis, prostate cancer (PCa), bladder cancer, bladder calculi, urethral stricture disease |
| **Which do you suspect?** | PCa with bony metastasis |
| **Why?** | African American male over age of 60 (both risk factors for PCa) presenting with bladder outlet obstruction symptoms (decreased stream strength, increased urinary frequency, sense of incomplete voiding) with or without UTI and pyuria with back pain (to rule out bone metastasis), weight loss (to rule out underlying malignancy), and hematuria is highly suspicious of metastatic PCa. |
| **What do you expect to find on rectal exam?** | Firm, nodular, or irregular prostate |
| **How is this different from the rectal exam with BPH?** | BPH typically has a smooth, symmetrically enlarged prostate with a rubbery consistency |
| **What labs should you order and why?** | Chem 8 (to rule out increased creatinine and renal insufficiency), CBC (to rule out anemia or leukocytosis), PSA (increased in most PCa), serum alkaline phosphatase (increased with bony metastasis) |
| **Does a normal PSA value rule out prostate cancer?** | No, but it makes the diagnosis less likely |
| **What increase in PSA is strongly correlated with prostate cancer?** | A PSA level 3–4 times the normal value |
| **If the alkaline phosphatase comes back elevated, does this confirm bone disease?** | No, it could have come from the liver |
| **What lab test can differentiate bone from liver alkaline phosphatase?** | Heat fractionization of alkaline phosphatase |

| | |
|---|---|
| **What result is consistent with bony mets?** | Decreased alkaline phosphatase with heat (bone burns liver lives) |
| **PSA comes back 6× normal (consistent with PCa). What diagnostic test should you order next?** | Ultrasound with biopsy |
| **What histologic diagnosis do you expect?** | Adenocarcinoma, because it is the most common type |
| **Prostate adenocarcinoma is diagnosed. What additional tests should be ordered because metastasis is suspected because of complaints of bone pain?** | Bone scan (for bone metastasis) and CT or MRI (metastatic lymphadenopathy) |
| **What is the treatment for** | |
|     **Men under 70 (this patient is 64)?** | Radical prostatectomy and radiation |
|     **Men over 70?** | Conservative or palliative therapy |
| **What additional therapy may be beneficial in late-stage disease?** | Antiandrogen therapy (diethylstilbestrol) or castration |
| **What tumor marker test should be ordered periodically to screen for cancer recurrence?** | PSA |
| **Does an elevated PSA indicate recurrence?** | Possibly, but it also could be BPH |

## CASE 6

*A 50-year-old male presents with painless lymphadenopathy in the neck and mild hepatosplenomegaly.*

| | |
|---|---|
| **What differential diagnosis are you considering?** | Throat infection, dental abscess, cat-scratch fever, lymphoma [Hodgkin lymphoma and non-Hodgkin lymphoma (NHL)], AIDS/HIV infection |

| | |
|---|---|
| **What's number one on your differential?** | Lymphoma |
| **Why?** | Painless lymphadenopathy with mild hepatosplenomegaly with no other infectious signs or symptoms is highly suggestive of lymphoma. |
| **Would your level of suspicion change if HSM were absent?** | No |
| **What basic labs should be ordered?** | CBC, Chem 8, LFT, coags (PT, PTT, and INR), ESR, LDH |
| **What results may be found in NHL?** | Mild anemia, elevated LDH, and ESR |
| **What diagnostic test should you order?** | Tissue biopsy |
| **Biopsy reveals low-grade lymphoma with malignant expansion of B cells (more common than T cell) and no Reed-Sternberg cells were present. What's your diagnosis?** | NHL |
| **What additional workup is required?** | CT scan, bilateral bone marrow biopsy, and aspiration to stage the disease |
| **Do you expect advanced disease?** | No, because there are no B symptoms (fever, chills, night sweats, and weight loss) |
| **Imaging and bone marrow biopsy support localized neck disease. What's your treatment?** | Chemotherapy, prednisone, and radiation (owing to localized disease) |
| **Name the common chemotherapy regimens for**<br>    **Low-grade lymphoma** | Chlorambucil or cyclophosphamide and prednisone |

| | |
|---|---|
| **Intermediate and high-grade lymphomas** | CHOP (cyclophosphamide, doxorubicin, vincristine, and prednisone) |
| **When should stem cell or autologous bone marrow transplant be considered?** | In patients who relapse following initial treatment with chemotherapy |

## ANEMIAS

### CASE 7

*A 65-year-old male with history of mild aortic stenosis calls the clinic to schedule an office visit for progressive fatigue and lethargy over the last 3 months. The appointment is scheduled, but before seeing the patient you request he go to the lab for some basic tests.*

| | |
|---|---|
| **What two tests should you order?** | CBC (to rule out anemic) with differential and TSH (to rule out hypothyroid) |
| **Hg 9, MCV 73, TSH 7; what's your diagnosis?** | Microcytic anemia |
| **What's the differential diagnosis for microcytic anemia?** | Iron deficiency (GI bleed most common, menstruation, genitourinary, hookworm), anemia of chronic disease, decreased iron absorption (postgastrectomy and celiac disease), increased iron demand (pregnancy), thalassemia trait or syndrome, other hemoglobinopathies, sideroblastic anemia, chronic renal failure, lead poisoning |
| **Which do you suspect in this patient?** | GI blood loss most likely secondary to arteriovenous malformations (AVMs) |
| **Why?** | Aortic stenosis is associated with AVMs |
| **What signs of iron deficient anemia may be evident on physical exam?** | Glossitis, koilonychias ("spoon nails"), and angular stomatitis |

**What basic test can be done at the bedside to support GI blood loss?**

Stool guaiac test (tests for occult blood)

**Hemoccult test is positive (GI blood loss is confirmed). What additional labs should be ordered to diagnose iron deficient anemia?**

Serum iron, ferritin, iron saturation, and total iron binding capacity (TIBC)

**What results do you expect in iron deficient anemia?**

    **Serum iron**

Low

    **Ferritin**

Low

    **Percent iron saturation**

Low

    **TIBC?**

High

**What test would confirm the diagnosis but is rarely done?**

Bone marrow biopsy revealing decreased or absent iron stores

**What diagnostic procedure should be done in this patient with GI blood loss and iron deficient anemia?**

Colonoscopy and, if negative, upper endoscopy

**What is the treatment?**

Correct underlying cause, and oral iron replacement therapy with ferrous sulfate or gluconate

## CASE 8

*A 37-year-old male with history of alcoholism compliant with AA and Crohn disease s/p ileal resection 3 years ago for SBO presents to your office complaining of getting tired at half his usual running distance. He is concerned that he may have steroid myopathy, which was suggested by an internet health website.*

**What are you more concerned about?**

$B_{12}$ or folate deficiency

**Why?**

Fatigue with exercise intolerance is a symptom of anemia, possibly from ileal resection causing $B_{12}$ deficiency or alcoholism (decreased intake) causing folate deficiency

**What other risk factors exist for**

**Folate deficiency?**

Increased demand (pregnancy, hemolytic anemia), malabsorption, and drugs (e.g., ethanol, methotrexate, azathioprim, trimethoprim, phenytoin, and sulfasalazine)

**$B_{12}$ deficiency?**

Pernicious anemia, gastrectomy, pancreatic insufficiency, ileal disease or resection, intestinal bacterial overgrowth and parasites

**Which deficiency are patients at greater risk of developing owing to lower body reserves?**

Folate deficiency

**How long would it take to develop a $B_{12}$ deficiency?**

Years

**Which deficiency is most likely in this patient?**

$B_{12}$ due to ileal resection

**Labs from 6 months ago reveal mild anemia and macrocytosis. What's the differential diagnosis for macrocytosis?**

Alcohol abuse, reticulocytosis, vitamin $B_{12}$ deficiency, folic acid deficiency, liver disease, hypothyroidism, marrow aplasia, myelofibrosis

**What's the basic workup for macrocytosis in a patient with unclear risk factors?**

CBC with differential and smear, $B_{12}$, folate, reticulocyte count, thyroid and liver function studies, retic

**What tests should be done in this patient?**

CBC with differential and smear, $B_{12}$, folate

| | |
|---|---|
| **What finding on peripheral smear supports the diagnosis of B$_{12}$ or folate deficiency?** | Presence of hypersegmented neutrophils |
| **How is the diagnosis made?** | Increased MCV with a low folate or vitamin B$_{12}$ level |
| **Lab workup confirms macrocytic anemia with low B$_{12}$ and hypersegmented neutrophils on smear diagnostic of B$_{12}$ deficiency. What additional test could determine the cause of the B$_{12}$ deficiency?** | Schilling test |
| **Should this patient be treated?** | Yes |
| **Why?** | To minimize risk of developing signs or symptoms of vitamin B$_{12}$ deficiency |
| **What are they?** | Neurologic manifestations of decreased vibratory and positional sense, ataxia, paresthesias, confusion, and dementia |
| **What is the therapy for his vitamin B$_{12}$ deficiency?** | Intramuscular (IM) vitamin B$_{12}$ |
| **If he resumes drinking and develops folate deficiency, what would be the therapy?** | Oral or IV folic acid and alchohol abstinence |

## CASE 9

*A 54-year-old male with history of DJD, BPH s/p treatment of UTI with bactrim 3 months ago presents complaining of fatigue, dyspnea on exertion, easy bruising, and epistaxis. He denies any chest pain, fever, chills, abdominal pain, or signs of GI blood loss. On physical exam skin pallor appreciated as well as dry blood in both nares and multiple ecchymosis on the arms. The heart is regular with no murmur rubs or gallops, and the chest is clear to auscultation bilaterally.*

| | |
|---|---|
| **What is the single most important lab test to order?** | CBC |
| **Why?** | Because low platelets and hemoglobin could explain his symptoms on presentation |
| **CBC reveals pancytopenia. What's the next simple lab test?** | Peripheral blood smear |
| **Smear reveals a paucity of platelets, red blood cells, granulocytes, monocytes, and reticulocytes. What's the next best test?** | Bone marrow aspiration |
| **Marrow is hypocellular. What's your differential diagnosis?** | Acquired aplastic anemia, inherited aplastic anemia (Fanconi's anemia), myelodysplastic syndromes, acute myelogenous leukemia |
| **Which is most likely in this patient given the history, presentation, and diagnostic tests?** | Acquired aplastic anemia |
| **What are the most common causes of aplastic anemia?** | Idiopathic about 50%; drugs are the second leading cause |
| **What risk factor was present in this patient?** | Bactrim (contains sulfa, which has been associated with aplastic anemia) |
| **What are some other risk factors associated with conditions for acquired aplastic anemia?** | Viral illness [hepatitis, Epstein-Barr virus, cytomegalovirus (CMV)], drugs (e.g., acetazolamide, chloramphenicol, penicillamine), or radiation |
| **How is aplastic anemia diagnosed?** | Pancytopenia with a normal MCV and peripheral blood smear with hypocellular bone marrow biopsy |
| **Why does it occur?** | Failure of the bone marrow stem cells |

| **What replaces the normal hemopoietic cells?** | Fat |
| --- | --- |

| **What is the treatment?** | Discontinue offending drugs, RBC and platelet transfusions as needed, and bone marrow transplant |
| --- | --- |

| **What is the therapy for patients unable to receive a BMT?** | Immunosuppressive therapy with cyclosporine, glucocorticoids, and antithymocyte globulin |
| --- | --- |

| **What are the indications for empiric broad-spectrum antibiotics?** | Fever and neutropenia |
| --- | --- |

## CASE 10

*A 45-year-old male presents with fatigue, dyspnea on exertion, and microcytic anemia.*

| **What is your differential diagnosis for microcytic anemia?** | Iron deficiency, anemia of chronic disease, sideroblastic anemia, thalassemia |
| --- | --- |

| **What labs tests should you order to narrow the differential diagnosis?** | Ferritin, serum iron, TIBC, and RDW |
| --- | --- |

**Using the table, quiz yourself on the expected values for each disease state listed.**

| Disease | Ferritin | Iron | TIBC | RDW |
| --- | --- | --- | --- | --- |
| Iron deficiency | ↓ | ↓ | ↑ | ↑ |
| Chronic disease | Nl/↑ | ↓ | ↓ | N |
| Sideroblastic anemia | N/↑ | ↑ | Nl | Nl |
| Thalassemia | Nl/↑ | Nl/↑ | Nl/↓ | Nl/↑ |

| | |
|---|---|
| **The labs come back with normal ferritin, TIBC, and red cell distribution width (RDW) with low serum iron. What's the most likely diagnosis?** | Sideroblastic anemia |
| **What risk factors for sideroblastic anemia should you ask about?** | Drugs (e.g., isoniazid, chloramphenicol), chronic alcoholism, lead poisoning, malignancy, and chronic inflammation, infection, or myelodysplastic syndrome |
| **How will you confirm the diagnosis?** | Bone marrow aspirate |
| **What diagnostic feature will be present?** | Ringed sideroblasts |
| **What causes sideroblastic anemia?** | Failure of the RBC to incorporate iron into the heme molecule, resulting in deposition of a "ring" of granules around the RBC nucleus (called ringed sideroblast in the bone marrow) and hypochromic anemia |
| **What is the treatment?** | Supportive, with transfusions as necessary, and treat any underlying causes |
| **What are patients at risk of developing despite therapy?** | Acute leukemia or complete bone marrow failure if it is caused by myelodysplastic syndrome |

## CASE 11

A 22-year-old healthy woman of Mediterranean descent arrives for her first prenatal visit and is found to have a hemoglobin of 9, MCV of 60, RDW 28, retic 8%. She is diagnosed with microcytic anemia. She denied excess menstrual bleeding, weight loss, or change in stool color, character, or frequency. On physical exam mild splenomegaly is appreciated and guaiac test is negative for occult blood. The remainder of the physical exam is normal.

**What diagnoses are you considering?**

Iron deficiency, thalassemia, or sideroblastic anemia

**What additional labs should be ordered?**

Iron panel, which includes serum iron, transferrin, and ferritin

**The iron workup is normal. What's the next step?**

Peripheral smear

**Smear reveals basophilic stippling, target cells. What diagnosis does this suggest?**

β-thalassemia

**What risk factor did she have for β-thalassemia?**

Mediterranean descent

**What other risk factors are there for β-thalassemia?**

African, Middle Eastern, Indian, or Asian descent

**Name the most common adult thalassemia.**

β-thalassemia minor (β-chain mutation)

**What other disease is β-thalassemia minor most often confused with?**

Iron deficient anemia as a result of the microcytosis

**You suspect β-thalassemia minor. What test and results will confirm your diagnosis?**

Hemoglobin electrophoresis showing increased levels of fetal hemoglobin and hemoglobin A2

**What is the treatment for β-thalassemia minor?**

Supportive, no specific treatment required

**What causes β-thalassemia?**

A genetic mutation in one of the globin genes resulting in failure to produce one of the globin chains

**Why do the defective adult hemoglobin molecules hemolyze?**

Failure to produce adequate quantities of one of the globin chains creates a surplus of the other. These additional globin chains then precipitate, forming Heinz bodies in the RBC, and destabilize the membrane, causing hemolysis.

| | |
|---|---|
| **What disease is β-thalassemia partially protective for?** | Malaria |

## CASE 12

*A 17-year-old male with history of sickle cell disease presents to the ER with acute onset of fever, malaise, chest pain, and shortness of breath after hiking at low altitudes.*

| | |
|---|---|
| **What's your diagnosis?** | Sickle cell disease crisis with probable acute chest syndrome |
| **How does sickle cell crisis often present?** | Fever, malaise, and a painful vaso-occlusive crisis in the back, ribs, and extremities lasting for several days |
| **When should you consider acute chest syndrome?** | Any sickle cell disease patient complaining of shortness of breath or chest pain |
| **What causes sickle cell disease?** | A single amino acid substitution on the β-chain of globin in the hemoglobin molecule |
| **How does this affect the RBC?** | It polymerizes ("sickles") in the deoxygenated state. |
| **Who is at risk?** | Homozygous S patients |
| **What most likely triggered this patient's attack?** | Dehydration secondary to hiking long distances |
| **What else can precipitate it?** | Fever, infection, and pregnancy |
| **What labs should you order to support the diagnosis of sickle cell crisis?** | CBC, reticulocyte count, MCV, unconjugated bilirubin, LDH, haptoglobin |
| **What lab values do you suspect**<br>**In general?** | Low hemoglobin (5–10 g/dL) with an increased reticulocyte count; MCV may be slightly increased |

**With hemolysis?**

Increased unconjugated bilirubin and LDH, low serum haptoglobin

**What findings on peripheral smear would support the diagnosis?**

Sickle-shaped RBCs with or without Howell-Jolly bodies (indicates functional asplenia)

**What additional radiographic study and lab test should be ordered on this patient as a result of his pulmonary symptoms?**

CXR and ABG to support the diagnosis of acute chest syndrome

**What are you looking for in the CXR and ABG?**

Pulmonary infiltrates and hypoxia

**The above labs and studies support sickle cell crisis with acute chest syndrome. Do you need to confirm the diagnosis before treating?**

No, the patient came in with the diagnosis and has a laboratory profile consistent with the disease; waiting for the definitive test would only delay treatment.

**What test would confirm the diagnosis made in the past?**

Hemoglobin electrophoresis depicting large numbers of hemoglobin S molecules (heterozygotes have both Hg A and S)

**What's your treatment for Sickle cell crisis?**

IV hydration, analgesics (narcotics), folate supplements, red blood cell transfusions as needed, and antibiotics if infection suspected

**Acute chest syndrome?**

Oxygen and empiric antibiotics

**What is the preventative treatment?**

Oral fluids to prevent dehydration and hypoxia, folic acid supplements, vaccinations (pneumococcal, hepatitis B, and influenzae), and yearly ophthalmologic exams

**What is a common complication of chronic sickling?**

Functional asplenia from repeated splenic infarctions

| | |
|---|---|
| **What infectious organisms are patients with functional asplenia at risk for?** | Encapsulated organisms (e.g., pneumococcus and hemophilus influenzae) and *Salmonella* |

## CASE 13

*A 52-year-old women with history of HTN, rheumatoid arthritis, DJD, and congestive heart failure (CHF) presents to the clinic after being discharged from the ER for fatigue and mild dyspnea on exertion. The discharge diagnosis reads normocytic anemia with no evidence of acute GI blood loss. Follow-up was recommended with you as her primary care physician. You review the chart and note that she had a screening colonoscopy 2 years ago which was negative and has had negative occult blood tests and mild anemia in the past with an Hg of 10. Her Hg now per ER records was 9.2.*

| | |
|---|---|
| **What defines normocytic anemia?** | MCV between 80 and 100 |
| **What's the differential diagnosis for normocytic anemia?** | Hemolysis, aplastic anemia, acute hemorrhage, renal failure, myelophthisis, combined microcytic and macrocytic anemia (e.g., iron and folate deficiency), endocrine disorders (hypothyroidism, gonadal dysfunction, adrenal insufficiency), anemia of chronic disease (secondary to connective tissue disorders, infection, cancer), bone marrow failure, and lead poisoning |
| **Which is most likely in this patient?** | Anemia of chronic disease (ACD) |
| **Which risk factors does she have for it?** | Long-standing inflammatory diseases (rheumatoid arthritis), autoimmune disorders (rheumatoid arthritis) |
| **Name 2 other risk factors that should be considered.** | Malignancy and chronic infection |
| **What labs should you order to support your diagnosis of ACD?** | CBC, serum iron, TIBC, ferritin |

**What lab values are consistent with ACD?**

**CBC**                                  Normochromic normocytic anemia

**Serum iron**                          Low

**TIBC**                                 Low

**Ferritin**                             Normal or increased (because it is an acute-phase reactant)

**How is ACD diagnosed?**          Underlying chronic disease with the above associated lab values

**What causes ACD?**               Decreased delivery of iron to developing erythroblasts, decreased erythropoietin with respect to degree of anemia, and impaired bone marrow response to erythropoietin

**What is the treatment?**          Correct underlying disease if possible (are her DM, DJD, and RA optimally managed?) and consider erythropoietin therapy

**Which four disease states may benefit from erythropoietin therapy?**          Chronic renal insufficiency, chronic infection, chronic inflammatory diseases, and anemia after chemotherapy treatment

## CASE 14

*A 23-year-old male football player with personal and family history of bleeding problems presents to the ER with pain and loss of function in his right knee after a game with marked edema and effusion of the knee with decreased range of motion. No bony tenderness is found; ligament stress tests are negative.*

**What's your differential diagnosis?**          Fracture, severe strain or sprain, hemarthrosis secondary to hemophilia

**Which is most likely?**          Hemophilia

**Why?**

Patient and family have history of bleeding disorder, and hemarthrosis can occur in these patients, especially if playing contact sports.

**How does hemophilia often present?**

With painful spontaneous bleeding into the joints (hemarthrosis) or with prolonged posttraumatic or postoperative bleeding

**Name the 2 most common hemophilias and their respective deficiency.**

Hemophilia A (factor VIII deficiency) and hemophilia B (factor IX deficiency)

**What causes hemophilia?**

A hereditary bleeding defect characterized by a deficiency of specific plasma clotting proteins required for blood coagulation

**What is the hereditary pattern?**

X-linked (male offspring are often affected while female offspring are carriers)

**What imaging test should be done in this patient?**

X-ray of the left knee to rule out fracture

**X-ray shows a joint effusion but no fracture. What lab tests should you order?**

CBC, PTT, PT, fibrinogen, and bleeding time

**What associated lab values do you expect to find?**

Most often, patients have a prolonged PTT with normal PT, fibrinogen level, and bleeding time.

**Labs and presentation are consistent with hemophilia. What diagnostic test should you order next?**

Factor specific assay

**What is diagnostic of Hemophilia A?**

Factor VIII (decreased)

**Hemophilia B?**

Factor IX (decreased)

**What is your treatment?**

Replace deficient factor, avoid platelet-inhibiting drugs (e.g., NSAIDS), and recommend patient play noncontact sports

CASE 15

*A 21-year-old college student presents with complaints of heavy menstrual bleeding throughout her life, frequent epistaxis, and an odd rash on her lower extremities after taking aspirin. Upon chart review you note in the family history that the patient's mother required blood transfusions with her pregnancy.*

| | |
|---|---|
| **What's your differential diagnosis?** | Thrombocytopenia and von Willebrand disease (vWD) |
| **Which do you suspect?** | vWD |
| **How can vWD disease present?** | Mucocutaneous bleeding (e.g., menorrhagia, GI bleeding, gingival bleeding, epistaxis, and easy bruising) and soft tissue bleeding with hemarthrosis |
| **What labs should you order?** | CBC, PT, PTT, bleeding time (assesses platelet function) |
| **What do you expect to find with the** | |
| **CBC?** | Microcytic anemia due to chronic blood loss |
| **PT?** | Normal |
| **PTT?** | Prolonged |
| **Bleeding time?** | Prolonged |
| **Labs are consistent with vWD. What test will confirm the diagnosis?** | Low vWF antigen, abnormal ristocetin cofactor activity, and abnormal ristocetin-induced platelet aggregation |
| **vWD is diagnosed. What causes it?** | An autosomal dominant coagulation disorder characterized by decreased levels of von Willebrand factor (vWF) leading to decreased adherence of platelets to injured vessel walls and decreased stability of factor VIII in the plasma |

**What is your therapy?**

Factor VIII or cryoprecipitates that contain vWF concentrates

**What may be useful in the future if she needs surgery?**

DDAVP

**What does DDAVP do?**

Increases secretion of vWF from Weibel-Palade bodies in the endothelium

# 7    Neurology

## INFECTIOUS DISEASES OF THE CENTRAL NERVOUS SYSTEM

### CASE I

*A 32-year-old female with asthma, recurrent paranasal sinus infections, and congenital heart defect visits her ENT doctor complaining of headache, stiff neck, and right arm weakness.*

| | |
|---|---|
| **What's your differential diagnosis?** | Brain abscess, rapidly growing brain tumors, meningitis, encephalitis, and subarachnoid hemorrhage |
| **Which do you suspect?** | Brain abscess |
| **Why?** | Paranasal sinus infections and congenital heart defects are both risk factors for brain abscess. |
| **Name a few other risk factors for brain abscess** | Dental procedures, artificial heart valves, recent infection, paranasal sinus infections, and pneumonia |
| **What tests should be included in the workup?** | Lumbar puncture, blood and throat cultures, chest x-ray (CXR), CT of head, cardiac ECHO in addition to routine chemistry, CBC, and Coagulation time (coags) |
| **What are you looking for by ordering the following?** | |
| LP | Meningitis (CSF shows pleocytosis, low glucose, elevated protein) |
| **Blood and throat cultures** | Causative organisms |
| **CXR** | Pneumonia |
| **CTH** | Focal brain masses, abscess, evidence of meningeal swelling |

| | |
|---|---|
| **Cardiac ECHO** | Valve vegetations and congenital heart defects |
| **CBC** | Leukocytosis |
| **Chem 8** | Check creatine to rule out renal insufficiency, assess electrolytes |
| **Coags** | Rule out coagulopathy due to likelihood of diagnostic invasive procedures |
| **What are the radiographic findings with a brain abscess?** | Ring-enhancing lesion |
| **What is the treatment?** | |
| **Medical** | IV antibiotics and sometimes intraventricular antibiotics, steroids to reduce mass effect and edema |
| **Surgical** | Ventricular drain to reduce acute intracranial pressure with surgical excision of abscess if antibiotics and drain fail |
| **What additional therapy is required?** | Treat source of infection if identified |

## CASE 2

*A 22-year-old previously healthy male is brought to the ER by his mother after displaying bizarre behavior. About 1 week ago, this reserved young man was excessively happy, slept little, and was calling all his friends to go out and meet women. A few days later he complained of a fever and headache with nausea and vomiting. Now he is lethargic and has difficulty speaking.*

| | |
|---|---|
| **What's your differential diagnosis?** | Viral or bacterial encephalitis, brain abscess, subdural empyema, brain tumors, subdural hematoma |
| **Which is most likely?** | Viral encephalitis |
| **Which virus?** | Herpes simplex virus |

| | |
|---|---|
| **What are the clues?** | Bizarre behavior followed by headache, fever, nausea, and vomiting with progressive lethargy, confusion, focal neurologic findings |
| **What are the risk factors?** | Usually spontaneous, neonates may be exposed in birth canal of infected mothers |
| **What's in your diagnostic workup?** | Chem 8, CBC PT, INR, CT head (or MRI), lumbar puncture for CSF analysis |
| **What do you expect to find in HSV encephalitis?** | |
| **CBC** | Leukocytosis |
| **Coags** | Normal |
| **CT head** | Low-density, nonenhancing lesions in the temporal lobe |
| **CSF** | Excess WBCs (lymphocytes, monocytes), RBCs (because of hemorrhagic component), and increased protein with decreased or normal glucose |
| **What additional test is ordered to make the diagnosis?** | PCR for HSV DNA in the CSF |
| **How was it diagnosed before PCR?** | Brain biopsy |
| **What is the treatment?** | Acyclovir and anticonvulsants for seizures |

## CASE 3

*A 19-year-old college male with history of asthma, appendectomy, migraines, and splenectomy 3 years ago after a motor vehicle accident calls your office complaining of progressive headache, neck stiffness, and confusion.*

| | |
|---|---|
| **What should you tell him?** | Go to the ER. |
| **What's your differential diagnosis?** | Meningitis (bacterial and viral), encephalitis, brain abscess, subarachnoid hemorrhage, and cerebral vasculitis |
| **What do you suspect?** | Bacterial meningitis |
| **How does it commonly present?** | Headache, neck stiffness, photophobia, and change in mental status |
| **What causes the symptoms?** | Inflammation of the meninges |
| **What risk factor for bacterial meningitis does he have?** | Splenectomy (defect in humoral immunity) |
| **What type of bacteria?** | Encapsulated bacteria (*Streptococcus pneumoniae, Neisseria meningitidis, Haemophilus influenzae*) |
| **What physical findings are suggestive of the meningitis (viral and bacterial)?** | Fever, nuchal rigidity, mental status abnormalities, focal neurologic findings (e.g., seizures) |
| **What are signs of meningeal irritation on physical exam?** | Brudzinski and Kernig signs |
| **Describe them.** | |
| **Brudzinski sign** | Neck flexion while supine leads to involuntary hip and knee flexion |
| **Kernig sign** | Knee extension with a flexed hip produces pain |
| **What type of meningitis is suggested by a petechial rash on physical exam?** | *Neisseria meningitidis* |
| **How is bacterial meningitis diagnosed?** | Lumbar puncture with CSF analysis |

**What results do you expect with**

    **Bacterial meningitis?**

Increased WBC with high polymorphonuclear cells, high protein, low glucose

    **Aseptic meningitis (nonbacterial, viral)?**

High lymphocytes, normal or slightly elevated protein, normal glucose

**What additional CSF test should be done before treatment?**

Gram stain and bacterial cultures

**What is the empiric treatment for bacterial meningitis in**

    **Adults and children over 3 months?**

Third-generation cephalosporin

    **Infants and neonates?**

Ampicillin and cefotaxime

**When are antibiotics adjusted?**

After results of Gram stain, culture, and drug sensitivity are reported

**What is the treatment in aseptic meningitis?**

Supportive therapy

## CASE 4

*An 8-year-old illegal immigrant boy from a third world country presents to the ER with his mother complaining of severe headache, stiff neck, and inability to move right arm. The mother informs you that he did not receive all his vaccinations prior to entering the United States.*

**What's your differential diagnosis?**

Meningitis, brain neoplasm, brain abscess, poliomyelitis

**Which is most likely considering lack of complete immunizations?**

Poliomyelitis

**How does it usually present?**

Fever, headache, stiff neck, muscle pain followed by asymmetric paralysis

**What is poliomyelitis?**

A viral infection of the spinal cord caused by poliovirus in the anterior horn and brain stem that causes cell destruction and produces the paralytic manifestations of poliomyelitis

**How does the virus enter the body?**

Fecal-oral contact

**What diagnostic tests should you order?**

Throat, stool, or CSF culture for poliovirus and/or polio-specific antibody test

**How do you differentiate poliomyelitis from Guillain-Barré syndrome (GBS) or acute inflammatory demyelinating polyneuropathy?**

Sensory symptoms are present in GBS but not in Polio.

**How is poliomyelitis treated?**

Supportive, including respiratory support if respiratory failure ensues

**How could this have been prevented?**

Oral Polio vaccination (OPV)

## DEGENERATIVE AND HEREDITARY DISEASES OF THE CENTRAL NERVOUS SYSTEM

### CASE 5

*A 45-year-old male presents to your clinic with a progressive illness over the last few months. First he noticed hand and feet weakness which is still present. Now he has muscle spasms and difficulty speaking which you appreciate. Physical exam reveals hand and foot weakness, atrophy. It is also positive for hyperreflexia and spasticity of both upper and lower extremities.*

**What diagnosis is most likely?**

ALS

**What other name for ALS is there?**

Lou Gehrig disease

| | |
|---|---|
| **How does it typically present?** | Combination of lower motor dysfunction (hand, foot weakness, atrophy, and muscle twitches) and upper motor neuron dysfunction (hyperreflexia) with or without brainstem involvement (dysarthria and dysphagia) |
| **What test is helpful in supporting the diagnosis?** | Electromyography and nerve conduction studies |
| **What imaging should be ordered to rule out spinal cord lesions?** | MRI of the cervical and thoracic spine |
| **How is the diagnosis made?** | Clinical pattern of both upper and lower motor neuron |
| **How is ALS treated?** | The antiglutamatergic drug riluzole increases life expectancy of ALS patients by 4-6 months. |
| **What is the overall prognosis?** | Without tracheostomy and ventilatory support, the life expectancy is less than 2 years after bulbar involvement. If there is predominantly spinal involvement, 5-year survival is approximately 20%. |

## CASE 6

*An 81-year-old male comes to the office with his wife. She apologizes for being late, but she says her husband needs frequent direction when driving to familiar places. He also repeats the same questions frequently and often does not remember what was said 5 minutes ago. But, if she talks about the old days, he can remember it in detail.*

| | |
|---|---|
| **What diagnosis do you suspect?** | Alzheimer disease |
| **What's in the differential diagnosis for Alzheimer disease?** | Pick disease (frontotemporal dementia), vascular dementia, Lewy body dementia and Cruetzfeldt-Jakob disease |

| | |
|---|---|
| **What test is helpful in ruling out Pick disease and vascular dementia?** | CT or MRI of head |
| **What findings on CT suggest diagnosis of Alzheimer disease?** | Cortical atrophy |
| **What clinical features if present would suggest Lewy body dementia?** | Gait/balance disorder, prominent hallucinations and delusions |
| **What test is helpful to rule out Creutzfeldt-Jakob disease?** | EEG |
| **Why suspect Alzheimer disease in this patient?** | Most common cause of dementia over age of 80 |
| **What symptoms may appear after short-term memory loss?** | Disorientation, depression, and agitation |
| **What lab tests should be performed?** | Complete blood cell count, serum electrolytes, glucose and BUN/creatinine, serum B12 levels, liver function tests, and thyroid function tests |
| **What are the clinical criteria used to diagnose Alzheimer disease?** | Dementia by clinical examination and documented by neuropsychological screens or tests, deficits in two or more areas of cognition, progressive worsening of memory and other cognitive functions, no disturbance of consciousness, onset between the ages of 40 and 90 years, and absence of systemic or CNS disorders which could account for the progressive deficits of memory and cognition |
| **How is a definitive diagnosis made?** | Neuropathologic examination at autopsy |

| | |
|---|---|
| **What is the treatment strategy?** | Cholinesterase inhibitors (donepezil, rivastigmine, or galantamine) |

## CASE 7

*A 62-year-old male with history of DJD, gout, BPH, and hyperlipidemia presents to the clinic with his wife after noting a tremor in his hand while resting. It goes away with intentional movement. As he walks toward you to the examining room, he appears to shuffle down the hallway and is slightly bent forward.*

| | |
|---|---|
| **What disease do you suspect he has?** | Parkinson disease |
| **What are the cardinal signs of Parkinson disease?** | Resting tremor, cogwheel rigidity, bradykinesia/akinesia, and postural reflex impairment |
| **How do you differentiate parkinsonian tremor from essential tremor?** | Parkinsonian tremor occurs at rest, while an essential tremor is a postural tremor seen when maintaining a posture or during an action |
| **What causes Parskinson disease?** | A neurodegenerative disease of unknown cause that results in loss of dopaminergic neurons in the substantia nigra pars compacta and the loss of their inputs to the striatum (globus pallidus and caudate nuclei) |
| **Which diagnostic tests are helpful?** | An MRI of the brain is usually done to rule out structural causes of parkinsonism. |
| **What are the pathologic findings in Parkinson disease?** | Loss of pigmented neurons in the substantia nigra pars compacta and appearance of Lewy bodies |
| **How is the diagnosis made?** | Clinically, and is considered definite if any three of the cardinal signs are present |

**What is the treatment?**

Levodopa combined with a peripheral DOPA-decarboxylase inhibitor (carbidopa in Sinemet, benserazide in Madopar) remains the single most effective medication.

## NEOPLASMS

### CASE 8

*A 55-year-old male with history of COPD from 60 pack years smoking comes to the ER after falling off his bike. He gradually became weaker on his right side, was not able to maintain his balance, and fell. Since arriving by ambulance, his right-sided facial, arm, and leg weakness has not improved.*

**What's your differential diagnosis?**

Brain tumors, stroke, resolving intracranial hemorrhage, brain abscess

**Which is most likely?**

Metastatic brain cancer from a primary lung cancer due to excessive smoking history

**How does a brain tumor typically present?**

Gradual decline in cognitive and intellectual ability, focal neurological signs, or seizures

**What is the most common primary brain neoplasm in Adults?**

Glioblastoma multiforme (malignant) and meningioma (benign)

**Children?**

Cerebellar astrocytoma and medulloblastoma

**What is the most common source of metastatic brain tumors?**

Lung cancer (most likely in this patient)

**What are the associated CT or MRI findings?**

Irregular lesions with surrounding edema or ring-enhancing lesions with or without edema or solid lesions with or without edema. Ventricules displace to opposite side. Hydrocephalus may be present.

| | |
|---|---|
| **What CT finding should raise suspicion of metastasis?** | Multiple brain lesions |
| **What is the treatment?** | Steroids to reduce edema, surgical excision or debulking followed by radiation and chemotherapy, anticonvulsants for seizure control |

## DEMYELINATING DISEASE

### CASE 9

*A 17-year-old previously healthy female presents to your office complaining of numbness in her right hand for the last 24 hours. She denies any trauma or headache preceding its onset. She does add that over the last month at various times her right field of vision was obscured for less than a day, and one morning she was unsteady on her feet. Because these symptoms went away over time, she did not feel it was necessary to see a doctor. But now she wants an answer to explain the bizarre symptoms.*

| | |
|---|---|
| **What do you think she has?** | Multiple sclerosis (MS) |
| **Why?** | Young female presenting with neurologic signs and symptoms separated by space and time |
| **What is MS?** | An acquired disease thought to be an autoimmune disease or viral in etiology that causes plaques of demyelination in the central nervous system |
| **Who gets multiple sclerosis?** | Women twice as often as men, with an age of onset from 15 to 50 years which peaks in the 20s |
| **How does MS commonly present?** | Optic neuritis with visual loss, limb weakness, sensory symptoms (such as numbness, parasthesia, and hypesthesia), cerebellar ataxia, nystagmus, and diplopia (due to cranial nerve VI palsy or internuclear ophthalmoplegia) |

**What findings on the following tests support the diagnosis of MS?**

**CSF**

Mild pleocytosis (5–50 lymphocytes) during acute attacks and increased protein with high IgG and oligoclonal bands which are persistent between attacks

**Electrophysiologic tests**

Evoked potential studies (visual evoked potentials, brainstem auditory evoked response, somatosensory evoked potentials) can be used to demonstrate subclinical lesions in CNS pathways.

**MRI**

Demyelinating plaques can usually be seen as areas of increased signal on T2 MRI, and active plaques may enhance.

**How is the diagnosis of MS made?**

Documenting multiple CNS lesions in time and space. This is often done by the clinical history and examination, and imaging.

**What is the typical course of MS?**

Acute onset of symptoms followed by a relapsing/remitting course with episodic exacerbation of new or recurrent symptoms and eventual burn-out of active disease

**What is the therapy for MS exacerbation?**

High-dose IV methylprednisolone may shorten acute exacerbation of MS symptoms, but has no long-term effect on the course of the disease.

**What other medications are there for multiple sclerosis?**

Two forms of β-interferon (β-interferon 1a or Avonex and β-interferon 1b or Betaseron) and glatiramer (Copaxone) are know as the ABC drugs and are effective in reducing the severity and frequency of exacerbation.

CASE 10

*A 55-year-old previously healthy male presents to the clinic with complaints of progressive bilateral weakness of the legs and arms 2 weeks after recovering from an upper respiratory tract infection. The symptoms began with fine paresthesias in the toes and fingertips, followed by lower extremity weakness that slowly progressed over days to involve the arms.*

| | |
|---|---|
| **What diagnosis are you considering?** | Guillain-Barré syndrome (GBS) |
| **What is the differential diagnosis of GBS?** | Chronic inflammatory demyelinating polyneuropathy, acute intermittent porphyria, central pontine myelinolysis, carcinomatous meningitis, and poliomyelitis |
| **How does GBS present?** | Weakness and sensory loss predominate, but ataxia, autonomic dysfunction (postural hypotension and arrhythmias), and back pain may also occur. |
| **What is the pathophysiology of GBS?** | An inflammatory demyelination of peripheral nerves, involving both sensory and motor nerves. Spinal roots are often involved early in the disease. |
| **What are the associated triggers of GBS?** | Roughly two-thirds of patients have upper respiratory infections or diarrheal illness 2 to 4 weeks prior to onset of weakness. |
| **What is the most commonly identified precipitant of GBS?** | *Campylobacter* infection |
| **What finding on the following support the diagnosis of GBS?** | |
| Physical examination | Weakness and sensory loss with early loss of deep tendon reflexes |
| **Nerve conduction studies** | Slowed conduction consistent with demyelination |
| **Cerebrospinal fluid** | Elevated protein |

**How is it diagnosed?**

Clinical presentations, physical examination, and nerve conduction studies

**What is the treatment strategy?**

Plasmapheresis or IVIg can shorten and reduce the severity of the acute phase.

**What are the possible complications of GBS?**

Respiratory compromise and arrhythmia

**What is the overall prognosis?**

Recovery begins within 4 weeks after progression ceases. 85% are ambulatory within 6 months, but >50% have some residual deficits, 5% remain severely disabled, and 16% are handicapped.

## DISEASES OF NEUROMUSCULAR JUNCTION AND MUSCLE

CASE 11

*A 32-year-old female presents to your office complaining of double vision, slurring her words, and difficulty swallowing food. These symptoms only appear after a long day or when very busy. For instance, after chewing a lot, she may have difficulty swallowing. And, last weekend while watching a tennis match her vision was blurred by the third set. But, if she rests the symptoms disappear until she resumes similar activity.*

**What disease do you suspect?**

Myasthenia gravis

**What is myasthenia gravis?**

An autoimmune disease with antibodies against nicotinic receptors at the neuromuscular junction; impairs normal transmission resulting in increased weakness and fatigue

**What risk factors does she have?**

Age and sex (most are young women in third decade of life)

**What are other known risk factors?**

Thymoma (15–40%), other autoimmune diseases (15%), and drugs such as penicillamine

**What are the common signs of myasthenia gravis?**

Fluctuating diplopia, dysarthria, dysphagia, extremity weakness, and respiratory difficulty. Symptoms are often diurnal, with rapid fatiguing and improvement after rest. Sensation and reflexes are preserved.

**What is the differential diagnosis for myasthenia gravis?**

Lambert-Eaton syndrome, botulism, and drug-induced myasthenia

**How is myasthenia gravis differentiated from Lambert-Eaton syndrome?**

Rapid repetitive stimulation or sustained muscle activity results in improved strength, not weakness as in MG.

**What tests should you order?**

Acetylcholine receptor antibodies, electromyography (EMG), CT chest, and edrophonium test (tensilon test)

**What results support the diagnosis?**
**Acetylcholine receptor antibodies**

Positive

**EMG**

Decrementing responses to repetitive stimulation on electromyography

**What test confirms the diagnosis?**

Administration of exogenous anti-cholinesterase such as edrophonium or neostigmine (tensilon test) provides temporary relief of symptoms.

**Why did you order a CT of the chest?**

Thymoma is associated with MG and must be excluded by chest CT

**What is the treatment strategy for**
**Moderate symptoms?**

Pyridostigmine, an acetylcholinesterase inhibitor that enhances transmission at the neuromuscular junction

**Severe symptoms?**

Immunosuppression with prednisolone, often with azathioprine

**When is surgery indicated?** Thymectomy should be performed if there is thymoma, and in patients with more than minimal symptoms under the age of 45 years. <u>Thymectomy is also used if there is residual thymus gland in older patients.</u>

## CASE 12

*A 3-year-old girl is brought to the clinic by her mother after the child woke up complaining of blurred vision, light sensitivity, and difficulty keeping his eyes open. The mother said she was fine yesterday when they were at the family farm eating some of grandma's home canned jams and picking apples from the trees.*

**What should you immediately suspect?** Botulism

**What is the differential diagnosis for botulism?** GBS, brainstem infarction, myasthenia gravis, tic paralysis, diphtheria, familial periodic paralysis, poliomyelitis

**How does botulism present?** First symptoms (12 hours to 10 days after ingestion) diplopia, ptosis, blurred vision, photophobia

**What classical early physical exam finding of botulism should you look for?** <u>Fixed dilated pupils</u>

**What was a major clue to the diagnosis?** Recently ingested home canned foods

**What is the pathophysiology of botulism?** Botulinum neurotoxin <u>blocks the release of acetylcholine from presynaptic terminals resulting in paralysis.</u>

**How does the toxin enter the body?** Botulinum toxin is released on death and autolysis of *Clostridium botulinum* in contaminated food. The <u>toxin is absorbed from the GI tract</u> into general circulation.

**What are the laboratory findings?** Normal cerebrospinal fluid and <u>abnormal EMG</u>

| | |
|---|---|
| **How is the diagnosis confirmed?** | By detection of the toxin in suspected food, feces, gastric contents, or by anaerobic culture for presence of *C. botulinum* |
| **What is the treatment?** | Cathartics (removes toxin from the GI tract) and botulism antitoxin |
| **What is the main complication of botulism?** | Respiratory failure requiring intubation and ventilator support in 40% of cases |

## CASE 13

*A 4-year-old boy is brought to the clinic with insidious onset of toe-walking, a waddling gait, and difficulty standing and walking. On physical exam you appreciate lumbar lordosis and large calves.*

| | |
|---|---|
| **What diagnosis should you suspect?** | Muscular dystrophy |
| **Which one is most common in children?** | Duchenne muscular dystrophy |
| **What's the other type?** | Becker muscular dystrophy |
| **What is the cause of Duchenne and Becker dystrophies?** | Abnormalities in the dystrophin gene |
| **How does Duchenne dystrophy present?** | Difficulty standing and walking, waddling gait with lumbar lordosis, shortening of the calf muscles with pseudohypertrophy by age 5 |
| **How does the disease progress?** | Most become wheelchair dependent by age 12 and subsequently develop progressive kyphosis and contractures. Death usually occurs in the third decade from respiratory compromise and infections. |
| **How does Becker dystrophy present?** | Similar but less severe symptoms and a later onset than Duchenne |

| | |
|---|---|
| **What lab result supports the diagnosis?** | Elevated creatine phosphokinase (CPK) |
| **How is the diagnosis confirmed?** | Muscle biopsy showing necrosis with variation in muscle fiber size and no dystrophin |
| **What are the treatment options in muscular dystrophy?** | Largely supportive with physical therapy, bracing, and pulmonary care |

### CASE 14

*A 38-year-old female with history of urinary tract infections and diabetes presents to your office complaining of difficulty climbing stairs and putting her groceries away in the kitchen cabinets. She has not had this problem before. While listening to her, you notice an erythematous rash around her eyes.*

| | |
|---|---|
| **What diagnosis do you suspect?** | Dermatomyositis |
| **What are the two most common forms of inflammatory myositis?** | Polymyositis (PM) and dermatomyositis (DM) |
| **How do you tell them apart?** | DM has a skin rash |
| **Describe the heliotrope rash associated with DM.** | Red violaceous eruption on the upper eyelids |
| **Describe Gottron sign associated with DM** | Symmetric erythematous violet colored eruption with scales over the extensor surfaces of the metacarpophalangeal and interphalangeal joints of the fingers |
| **Describe the weakness in PM and DM.** | Progressive symmetric weakness of proximal muscles of hips and shoulders, often with myalgia and muscle tenderness |
| **What lab values should be elevated?** | CPK and aldolase to establish the extent of muscle breakdown |

| | |
|---|---|
| **What special test will aid in making the diagnosis?** | EMG with an "irritative" myopathy pattern |
| **How is the diagnosis confirmed?** | A muscle biopsy that reveals necrosis, degeneration, regeneration, and an inflammatory cell infiltrate |
| **What additional workup needs to be done?** | Search for an underlying malignancy |
| **Why?** | An underlying malignancy is found in 15 to 25% of cases |
| **How is myositis treated?** | Prednisone with gradual taper once a response is obtained; treat underlying malignancy if found |

## VASCULAR DISEASES OF THE CENTRAL NERVOUS SYSTEM

### CASE 15

*A 72-year-old male with history of diabetes, COPD secondary to smoking, hypertension, CAD s/p CABG 6 years ago presents to the ER with right-sided weakness and dysarthria that began 6 hours ago. On physical exam you appreciate right-sided weakness and a strong bruit over the carotids.*

| | |
|---|---|
| **What should be in your differential diagnosis?** | Transient ischemic attack (TIA) stroke, amaurosis fugax (shade comes down over ipsilateral eye) indicating possible internal carotid stenosis |
| **What risk factors for atherosclerosis does he have?** | Atherosclerosis, smoking, hypertension, diabetes mellitus |
| **What additional risk factors are associated with atherosclerosis?** | Hypothyroidism, hyperuricemia, hypercholesterolemia, or hypertriglyceridemia |
| **What is the significance of the carotid bruit?** | Suggestive of significant carotid stenosis |

**What diagnostic tests should you order?**

    **Labs**                     Chem 8, CBC, PT/INR, CK-MB, and troponin

    **Imaging**             CT or MRI of head, duplex ultrasound of all 4 neck vessels or magnetic resonance arteriography, trans thoratic echocardiogram (TTE)

**Why 4 vessel ultrasound?**      Present and status of collateral circulation important to surgeon

**Why TTE?**              High incidence of coronary artery disease and MI in patients with severe carotid stenosis

**How do you detect emboli breaking off the carotid plaque?**     Transcranial doppler studies of the circle of Willis

**Additional studies if this patient was younger with a family history of stroke?**    Antithrombin III, anticardiolipins, serum homocysteine, factor V Leiden, protein C, protein S, sickle cell

**What is the medical treatment?**     Treat known risk factors, aspirin, aspirin plus dipyridamole, and clopidogrel

**What surgical treatment is available?**     Carotid endarterectomy if stenosis >50% lumen or if stenosis demonstrates ulcerated plaques

**Why surgery for ulcerated plaques?**     To remove source of platelet or thrombotic emboli

## CASE 16

*A 64-year-old male with history of HTN, Achilles tendon rupture, CAD s/p MI with abnormal LV function (akinetic portion of ventricle) presents to the ER in atrial fibrillation with left-sided hemiparesis and aphasia.*

**What's the most likely cause?**     Cardioembolic stroke

**How does cardioembolic stroke present?**

Any of the following: acute onset hemiparesis, hemianesthesia, impaired level of consciousness, decreasing level of consciousness (cerebral edema), loss of vision (homonymous hemianopia), loss of language (dysphasia or aphasia), neglect on paralyzed side (anosognosia autotopagnosia)

**What are his known risk factors?**

Atrial fibrillation and akinetic portion of LV from prior MI

**Name other risk factors predisposing to embolism.**

Diseased heart valves (rheumatic fever, bacterial endocarditis), recent MI with mural thrombosis, ventricular aneurysm, patent foramen ovale, artificial heart valves, ulcerated atheromatous plaques in ascending aorta or internal carotid artery

**What causes the stroke?**

Cerebral infarction and loss of neurologic function due to embolism of a cerebral artery

**What do you expect to find on neurologic examination?**

Hemiparesis or hemiplegia with flaccid limbs and depressed reflexes, and extensor plantar responses on affected side, gradual development of spasticity and increased reflexes on affected side after 72 hours

**What labs should you order?**

CBC, PT/INR, Chem 8, CK-MB, tropinin

**What tests should you order?**

Noncontrast CT scan of head to determine if ischemic or hemorrhage infarction and anatomic site, EKG, 2D echocardiogram, TTE, 4 vessel (carotid and vertebral arteries) duplex ultrasound (doppler and real time), cardiology consultation to rule out or detect associated heart disease (stroke patients have a high risk of MI)

**What is the treatment strategy in this patient with atrial fibrillation?**

Assume cardiac embolism and anticoagulate

| | |
|---|---|
| **When else is anticoagulation treatment warranted?** | If studies reveal source of embolism, i.e., valvular disease, PFO, mural thrombus, cerebral arteritis, recent MI |
| **When should anticoagulants be prescribed?** | Use anticoagulants—heparin followed by warfarin—in cases of proven embolus |
| **What tests should be ordered if patient is anticoagulated?** | Activated clotting time or partial thromboplastin time (PTT) for heparin therapy.<br><br>Prothrombin time (PT) with INR (international normalized ratio) for coumadin therapy |
| **What additional therapy is indicated for long-term prevention of recurrent stroke or MI?** | Treat atrial fibrillation; may need cardioversion and/or antiarrhythmic drugs. If present treat hypertension, diabetes mellitus, hyperlipidemia, hyperuricemia, hypothyroidism, obesity, tobacco abuse, alcoholism. |
| **When is surgical treatment indicated?** | Patent foramen ovale (PFO) or heart valve replacement |
| **What therapy is available for patients who cannot or refuse to take anticoagulation?** | Aspirin, aspirin plus dipyridamole, clopidogrel, or ticiopidine |

## CASE 17

A 72-year-old male with history of HTN, CAD s/p 3 vessel CABG 4 years ago, and TIAs presents to the ER after developing over 24 hours of a clumsy right hand and dysarthria. Because he had TIAs in the past he thought it would go away as long as he kept taking his aspirin. Preliminary MRI shows multiple small subcortical lesions.

| | |
|---|---|
| **What's your diagnosis?** | Lacunar stroke |
| **What is the usual presentation?** | Clumsy hand with dysarthria, dysphasia, or ataxia |

| | |
|---|---|
| **What causes it?** | Small vessel vasculopathy due to athero-sclerosis, arteriosclerosis, or embolism of terminal penetrating arteries |
| **What are the risk factors?** | Hypertension, atherosclerosis and dia-betes mellitus, and carotid artery stenosis |
| **What radiographic studies should be ordered?** | CT or MRI will show small localized lesions which may be cortical, subcortical, or located in deeper structures including the internal capsule, caudate nucleus putamen, brainstem, or cerebellum. |
| **What is the treatment?** | Treat underlying risk factors. Give aspirin or clopidogrel. |
| **Surgical treatment?** | Carotid endarterectomy in those patients with >50% stenosis to eliminate repeated embolism |
| **What is the prognosis with mild symptoms?** | Most have rapid improvement, but major stroke or MI is a risk factor. |

## CASE 18

*Your attending asks you to see a patient in the ER examining room who had a stroke and asks you to obtain a history from the patient and his wife and tell him where the lesion was without seeing the imaging reports.*

| | |
|---|---|
| **What are the main arteries to consider before walking into the room?** | Middle cerebral artery, anterior cerebral artery, posterior cerebral artery, and ver-tebrobasilar artery |
| **Recall common symptoms of stroke in** | |
| **Anterior cerebral artery** | Contralateral leg weakness and behav-ioral changes |
| **Middle cerebral artery** | Contralateral limb weakness (arm > leg) with sensory loss, homonymous hemi-anopsia, aphasia (dominant hemisphere involvement), sensory neglect or apraxia (nondominant hemisphere) |

| | |
|---|---|
| **Posterior cerebral artery** | Contralateral homonymous hemianopsia, sensory loss, thalmic pain, or involuntary movements |
| **Vertebrobasilar artery (unilateral occlusion)** | Ipsilateral cranial nerve abnormalities with contralateral weakness and sensory deprivation |
| **What imaging modalities will help you determine if it's ischemic or hemorrhagic?** | MRI or CT |
| **Which test is more likely to show signs of cerebral ischemia soon after a stroke?** | MRI |
| **What are the basics principles to treating strokes?** | Do not use antihypertensives in a patient with an evolving stroke (may further decrease cerebral blood flow); search for underlying causes (e.g., carotid embolism, carotid artery stenosis, hemorragic bleed), consider heparin in nonhemorragic evolving stroke, aspirin or plavix. |

## CASE 19

*A 64-year-old male with history of uncontrolled hypertension, atrial fibrillation on coumadin, hiatal hernia, and diverticulosis presents to the ER after a motor vehicle collision with sudden onset headache, nausea, vomiting followed by change in mental status.*

| | |
|---|---|
| **What most likely happened?** | Intracranial hemorrhage |
| **What are the pathologic changes prior to intracranial hemorrhage?** | Arteriolosclerosis of the penetrating vessels entering the brain leading to weakness of vessel walls and occasionally aneurysm formation (Charcot-Bouchard aneurysm) |
| **What risk factors does he have?** | Hypertension, anticoagulated (coumadin), trauma |
| **How might his symptoms advance?** | Stupor and coma |

| | |
|---|---|
| **What 3 things should you do first in the ER?** | (1) Establish airway<br><br>(2) Obtain coagulation profile (PT and PTT)<br><br>(3) Obtain head CT |
| **What are the associated findings in the spinal fluid?** | CSF can be clear unless there has been associated bleeding into the subarachnoid space. |
| **CT is diagnostic of intra-cerebral hemorrhage. What's the treatment?** | Control hypertension, maintain airway, and monitor the heart. Stabilize coagulation deficits, and lower intracranial pressure, if necessary. |

## CASE 20

*A 32-year-old medical resident with history of polycystic kidney disease and coarctation of the aorta presents after weight lifting with acute onset of severe headache with pain spreading to back of head and stiff neck. Later he developed nausea, vomiting, and confusion. Prior to this, the patient had a headache that was unresponsive to over-the-counter analgesics which had worked before. This is the worst headache of his life.*

| | |
|---|---|
| **What diagnosis is most likely?** | Subarachnoid hemorrhage (SAH) |
| **What are the causes of SAH?** | Ruptured saccular (Berry) aneurysm around the circle of Willis, trauma, bleeding diathesis, arteriovenous malformations, and illicit drug use (cocaine and amphetamine) |
| **Based on history, what cause do you suspect?** | Ruptured Berry aneurysm |
| **What were the clues?** | PCK and coarctation of aorta are both associated with Berry aneurysms. |
| **When does ruptured aneurysm occur?** | When patient is active, at work, exercising, or straining, but can occur at rest |

**How does a ruptured aneurysm present?**

Sudden onset severe headache (worst headache of their life) with pain spreading to occiput and neck, and nuchal rigidity

**What's the name for the headache that the patient had that was unresponsive to over-the-counter medications?**

Sentinel headache

**Is sentinel headache always a feature of saccular aneurysm?**

No, sentinel headache rarely indicates presence of aneurysm.

**What fundoscopic change might you find on physical exam?**

Papilledema can develop as early as 6 hours after rupture of aneurysm

**What labs should be included in the workup?**

CBC, PT, PTT, INR, and CMP

**What's the diagnostic test?**

CT head without contrast showing blood within the pia and arachnoid layers

**What's the therapy?**

IV narcotics for pain, diazepam for anxiety and seizure prophylaxis, surgery for drainage if easily accessible

**Prognosis of ruptured saccular aneurysm?**

30% die within 24 hours; 40% die within 7 days; 50% of survivors have second bleed; 60% die within 6 months.

## EPISODIC DISORDERS

CASE 21

*A 48-year-old female with history of drug abuse presents to the ER with uncontrollable jerking of the right arm for the last 5 minutes. She says this has never happened before.*

**What do you suspect?**

New onset of seizure

**What's in the differential diagnosis for seizure?**

Transient ischemic attack, migraine, metabolic derangements, transient global amnesia, paroxysmal movement disorders, pseudoseizures

**What are common causes of seizure in the various groups below?**

**Children**

Fever, CNS infections, and electrolyte abnormalities

**Adult**

Alcohol and drug withdrawal, electrolyte imbalance, trauma, eclampsia

**Elderly**

Trauma, brain cancer, CVA

**What types of seizures are there?**

Partial (simple and complex) and generalized (absence seizures, tonic-clonic, tonic, clonic, myoclonic, and atonic)

**How are simple and complex partial seizures similar?**

Both have focal motor or sensory deficits

**How are they different?**

Simple has no alteration in consciousness while complex does

**What type of seizure does this patient present with?**

Simple partial seizure

**What cause do you suspect?**

ETOH or drug withdrawal

**What labs should you order?**

CBC, chemistry studies for electrolytes, glucose, calcium, magnesium, uremia, and hepatic encephalopathy, and toxicology screen

**What diagnostic tests are helpful?**

EEG and MRI to locate focal abnormality

**Can simple seizures progress to something else?**

Yes, either type can evolve secondarily to generalized

**Describe the following types
of generalized seizures.**
**Absence (petit-mal)**

Brief loss of consciousness without
loss of muscle tone, aura, or postictal
confusion

**Tonic-clonic (grand-mal)**

Aura may occur before tonic contraction
with arched back followed by rapid alteration of muscle contraction and relaxation, postictal confusion and headache
common

**What's the workup?**

Same as partial seizure

**How are seizures treated?**

A single seizure of unknown cause,
or seizures secondary to specific or
treatable causes (febrile seizures,
alcohol withdrawal seizures, seizures
secondary to hypoglycemia, etc.) do
not require initiation of anticonvulsant
therapy.

**When is chronic anticonvul-
sant therapy warranted?**

Recurrent seizures

**Name commonly used drugs
of choice for**
**Simple partial, complex
partial, and generalized
tonic-clonic seizures**

Phenytoin, carbamazepine, and valproic
acid

**Absence, myoclonic, and
atonic seizures**

Valproic acid and ethosuximide

**When is surgery warranted?**

Seizures refractory to medical treatment

**What is status epilepticus?**

Continuing or recurring seizures without
complete recovery between attacks, last-
ing more than 20 minutes

**What type of seizure does it
occur with?**

Any type

| | |
|---|---|
| **What labs should you order?** | CBC, chemistry panel, anticonvulsant drug levels, and arterial blood gas should be sent STAT; also send a toxicology screen and do a finger stick for glucose. |
| **What's the medical therapy?** | IV fosphenytoin followed by IV lorazepam if seizures persist |
| **What's required if respiratory failure develops?** | Intubation |

# 8   Rheumatology

## GENERAL MUSCULOSKELETAL PROBLEMS

CASE 1

*A 40-year-old female with history of irritable bowel syndrome (IBS, a.k.a visceral hypersensitivity) presents with complaints of multiple areas of tender muscles, stiffness, generalized fatigue, and not sleeping well.*

| | |
|---|---|
| **What's your differential diagnosis?** | Muscle strain or sprain, fibromyalgia, hypothyroidism, psychogenic rheumatism, polymyalgia rheumatica, temporal arteritis |
| **Which is most likely?** | Fibromyalgia |
| **Why?** | Because she presents with the classic poorly localized muscle pain that spares the joints, stiffness, fatigue, nonrestorative sleep with an associated condition of IBS |
| **What other associated conditions are there?** | Tension headache and dysmenorrhea |
| **What physical exam findings do you expect to find?** | Bilateral tender points over the trapezius ridge, posterior cervical musculature, upper gluteal area, and trochanteric bursae |
| **What are the associated lab findings?** | Normal white blood cell count and erythrocyte sedimentation rate |
| **How is the diagnosis made?** | Clinical history and physical exam |
| **What is the treatment strategy?** | Tricyclic antidepressants, physical therapy, and aerobic exercise for muscle aches. No role for NSAIDs. |

## CASE 2

*A 20-year-old female presents 1 week after camping in Connecticut in July with a new rash (Figure 8-1) with low grade fever, headache, malaise, and myalgias.*

| | |
|---|---|
| **What is your differential diagnosis?** | Lyme disease, viral syndrome, juvenile rheumatoid arthritis |
| **Which is most likely?** | Lyme disease |
| **Why?** | Patient presents with classic rash of erythema chronicum migrans (bulls-eye appearance) 1 week after (onset often 7–10 days) camping in high prevalence area (Connecticut) during peak incidence time (May to August) with mild influenza-like symptoms |
| **Do all patients present like this 1 week after?** | No, some may only have the rash. |
| **What laboratory test should you order first?** | Enzyme-linked immunosorbent assay (ELISA) |
| **What additional test should you order if the ELISA test is positive?** | A Western blot to confirm because ELISA tests are often false-positives |

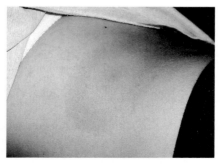

**Figure 8–1.**
*Source:* Goodheart HP. Goodheart's Photoguide of Common Skin Disorders, 2nd Ed. Philadelphia: Lippincott Williams & Wilkins, 2003.

| | |
|---|---|
| **Can ELISA and Western blot distinguish between active and previous infections?** | No |
| **How is the diagnosis made?** | Strong clinical suspicion (endemic area, tick bite, and rash) with positive ELISA and Western blot |
| **What causes lyme disease?** | The tick spirochete *Borrelia burgdorferi* |
| **What areas of the country have a high prevalence of this tick?** | Northeastern coastal states, the upper Midwest, and northern California |
| **What is the treatment?** | Oral doxycycline or amoxicillin and probenecid |
| **Why is it important to treat lyme disease?** | To prevent potential rheumatologic, cardiac, and neurologic complications |

## CASE 3

*A 62-year-old female with history of HTN and diabetes presents with progressive left-sided throbbing temporal headaches, scalp tenderness, and slight blurring of vision.*

| | |
|---|---|
| **What's your differential diagnosis?** | Temporal arteritis (TA), cerebral vascular accident, retinal detachment |
| **Which diagnosis is most likely?** | TA |
| **Why?** | |
| Age | Over 50 |
| Headache | Unilateral and temporal |
| Eyesight | Blurred |
| **What physical exam finding would support your diagnosis?** | Nodular, enlarged, tender, or pulseless temporal artery |

**Is this always present?** No

**What additional symptom is present in some patients and fairly specific for TA?** Jaw or tongue claudication with mastication

**What lab test should you order?** ESR

**What value supports the diagnosis of TA?** >50

**How is diagnosis confirmed?** Temporal artery biopsy

**What do you expect the pathology report to say?** Granuloma with giant multinucleated giant cells of the intima and media with disruption of the internal elastic lamina

**What causes TA (a.k.a. giant cell arteritis)?** A progressive inflammatory disorder of unknown etiology that affects mainly large cranial arteries, primarily the temporal artery

**What is the TA treatment?** High-dose oral prednisone (60 mg/daily) immediately without biopsy results with gradual tapering

**Why start treatment without biopsy confirmation?** To prevent irreversible blindness

**6 months later the same woman returns to clinic and is grateful to you for saving her vision, but complains of fatigue and difficulty with climbing stairs, getting out of bed in the morning, and combing her hair because of muscle pain and stiffness. What's your differential diagnosis?** Polymyositis/dermatomyositis, polymyalgia rheumatica, thyroid disease, viral myalgia or myopathy secondary to steroids, alcohol or electrolyte imbalance

**Which is most likely?** Polymyalgia rheumatica (PMR)

| | |
|---|---|
| **Why?** | It often coexists in patients with a history of TA and often presents in elderly patients over the age of 50. |
| **Why is polymyositis less likely?** | The patient complains of muscle pain and stiffness, not weakness. |
| **What labs should you order?** | CBC, TSH, ESR, CK, and aldolase |
| **What results would support your diagnosis of PMR?** | Anemia and elevated ESR |
| **How is PMR diagnosed?** | Clinically based on pain and stiffness (not weakness) in the shoulder and pelvic girdle area; fever, malaise, and weight loss may be present. |
| **What causes PMR?** | PMR is a chronic, intermittent, inflammatory disease of the large arteries. |
| **What's the treatment?** | Low-dose prednisone with gradual tapering |

## CASE 4

*A 48-year-old female with history of degenerative joint disease (DJD) and prolapsed bladder presents with progressive difficulty climbing stairs, combing her hair, and a new facial rash.*

| | |
|---|---|
| **What is this woman's main clinical problem?** | Proximal muscle weakness of the shoulder and pelvic girdle |
| **What's your differential diagnosis?** | Dermatomyositis, polymyositis, drug-induced or inflammatory myopathy, thyroid disease, systemic lupus erythematous, vasculitis |
| **Physical exam confirms 3/5 bilateral shoulder and pelvic girdle weakness and a heliotrope skin rash (bilateral raccoon eyes). What's the most likely diagnosis?** | Dermatomyositis |

| | |
|---|---|
| **What labs should you order to support your diagnosis?** | Elevated creatine phosphokinase and aldolase |
| **What additional test could you order?** | EMG |
| **What would you expect it to find?** | Muscle irritability, low-amplitude potentials, polyphasic potentials, and fibrillations |
| **How is the diagnosis confirmed?** | Muscle biopsy |
| **What do you expect the pathology report to say?** | Muscle cell degeneration with an inflammatory infiltrate, phagocytic debris, and perifascicular muscle fiber atrophy |
| **How would polymyositis be diagnosed?** | Identical to dermatomyositis without the heliotrope skin rash |
| **Describe the treatment strategy for both DM and PM.** | High-dose oral prednisone with taper to goal of normalizing muscle enzymes |

## CASE 5

*A 44-year-old woman with history of joint pains and DJD presents with complaint of her finger tips turning blue in cold weather and difficulty swallowing her food over the past month.*

| | |
|---|---|
| **What's your differential diagnosis for cyanotic fingers?** | Raynaud phenomenon, rheumatoid arthritis, progressive systemic sclerosis, SLE, Buerger disease |
| **Which is most likely given the brief history?** | Raynaud phenomenon |
| **Does her complaint of dysphagia broaden your differential from simply Raynaud to explain her symptoms?** | Yes |

**Why?**

Raynaud phenomenon and esophageal dysmotility are part of a limited form of systemic scleroderma called CREST syndrome

**What do the letters in CREST stand for?**

**C**alcinosis, **R**aynaud phenomenon, **E**sophageal dysmotility, **S**clerodactyly, **T**elangiectasias

**Who is at the greatest risk of developing CREST?**

Women in their third to fifth decade (this patient was female and 44)

**How may patients with CREST (limited scleroderma) commonly present early in the disease?**

Thick, tight, shiny skin, Raynaud phenomenon, and polyarthralgia (this patient had joint pain)

**How is the diagnosis made?**

Strong clinical suspicion, anticentromere antibodies

**What problems are associated with the antibody tests?**

Lack of sensitivity and (usually) specificity decreases their effectiveness in making the diagnosis.

**What is the pathogenesis behind CREST syndrome?**

Diffuse fibrosis of the skin and internal organs of unknown etiology

**What is the treatment strategy?**

Symptomatic and supportive because no definitive treatment is available

**What is the treatment for the following?**

    **Severe Raynaud phenomenon**

Vasodilating drugs (Ca channel blockers or prazosin)

    **Skin and periarticular changes**

Physical therapy

    **GI hypomotility (dysphagia)**

Aggressive gastroesophageal management, antibiotics for intestinal bacteria overgrowth, and prokinetic agents such as metoclopramide if significant gastroparesis develops

## CASE 6

*A 38-year-old female returns to your clinic for follow-up of low grade fever, fatigue, and malaise that was attributed to a viral illness and symptomatic therapy with acetominophen recommended. She now complains of joint pain, bright light sensitivity, nausea, and a rash on her face that is in the shape of a butterfly.*

| | |
|---|---|
| **What is most striking about her complaints?** | Multisystem involvement |
| **What is your differential diagnosis for multisystem complaints?** | HIV, systemic lupus erythematosus (SLE), scleroderma, rheumatoid arthritis, mixed connective tissue disease |
| **Which is most likely in her?** | SLE |
| **Why?** | Waxing and waning of multisystem complaints with fever, fatique, malaise, malar rash ("butterfly" skin rash), and photosensitivity is a common initial presentation for SLE. |
| **What causes it?** | Unknown, but autoantibodies to nuclear and other autoantigens are suspected |
| **Name other common presentations of SLE by organ system.** | |
|     **Musculoskeletal** | Arthralgias, myalgias, and arthritis |
|     **Central nervous system** | Seizures, psychosis, anxiety, and depression |
|     **Cardiac** | Pericarditis, myocarditis, endocarditis, and arrhythmias |
|     **Gastrointestinal** | Nausea, vomiting, anorexia, and abdominal pain |
|     **Vascular and hematologic** | Anemia, thrombocytopenia, lymphadenopathy, and splenomegaly |
|     **Immune** | Lymphadenopathy and splenomegaly |

| | |
|---|---|
| **Renal** | Impairment may be from associated vasculitis. |
| **When should the diagnosis be considered?** | When a young woman presents with multisystemic findings |
| **What serologic markers should you order?** | Antinuclear antibody, anti-double stranded DNA, and anti-Sm |
| **Which serologic tests are more specific?** | Anti-double stranded DNA and anti-Sm |
| **The diagnosis is made. What is your treatment for her?** | NSAIDs, hydroxychloroquine (for her dermatologic and musculoskeletal manifestations) |
| **Are steroids indicated in her case now?** | No |
| **When are steroids appropriate?** | For severe systemic symptoms (glomerulonephritis, severe CNS involvement, thrombocytopenia, and hemolytic anemia) and debilitating manifestations unresponsive to conservative treatment |

## DISORDERS OF THE BACK, SPINE, AND BONE

### CASE 7

*A 22-year-old male presents to your clinic complaining of low back pain after falling on his back while playing basketball.*

| | |
|---|---|
| **What's your brief differential diagnosis for low back pain?** | Lumbar strain, disk disease, vertebral fracture |
| **How do they commonly present?** | |
| **Strain** | Localized lower back pain without radiation (nerve root not involved) with regional tenderness, severe restriction of movements, and paraspinal muscle spasms on exam |

| | |
|---|---|
| **Lumbar disk disease** | Back pain with decreased mobility and compensatory posture. Pain will radiate to the groin and or leg (usually unilateral) if nerve root is compressed. |
| **Vertebral fractures** | Sudden onset of excruciating pain |
| **What are red flag symptoms of back pain?** | Bowel or bladder incontinence |
| **What level is involved if bowel or bladder symptoms are present?** | Conus medullaris or cauda equina |
| **What tests should be ordered if lumbar disk disease or vertebral fracture is suspected?** | X-ray or CT scan |
| **How are the various diagnoses made?** | Clinical presentation and x-ray or CT scan |
| **What is the treatment strategy for acute lower back pain?** | NSAIDs, bed rest, muscle relaxants, and surgical consult if radiographic studies reveal underlying pathology or red flag symptoms are present |
| **What additional medication should be prescribed without delay if red flag symptoms are present?** | IV steroids |

CASE 8

*A 17-year-old male with history of multiple admissions for heroin overdose presents to the ER complaining of dull back pain. He denies any recent trauma or history of back disease. Spinal tenderness, swelling, warmth, and erythema exist in the mid-thoracic region without radiation.*

| | |
|---|---|
| **What's in your differential diagnosis for back pain?** | Strain, disk disease, fracture, and osteomyelitis |

| | |
|---|---|
| **Which should be highest on your differential diagnosis for this patient?** | Osteomyelitis |
| **What causes it?** | An infection of the bone, usually caused by direct or hematogenous spread of bacteria from a wound or local infection |
| **Why do you suspect it in this patient?** | IVDA (strong risk factor), spinal tenderness and warmth on exam |
| **What other risk factors exist for osteomyelitis?** | Coexisting infections, age, diabetes, and immunodeficiency (HIV) |
| **What are other common presentations of osteomyelitis?** | Incapacitated or limping with dull pain over long bones (femur, humerus, tibia) |
| **What physical exam clues did this patient have for osteomyelitis?** | Point tenderness, swelling, warmth |
| **What additional findings are common?** | Systemic fever, erythema, effusion, decreased range of motion, and regional muscle spasms in the affected area |
| **What should you order?** **Labs** | White blood cell count, erythrocyte sedimentation rate, c-reactive protein, and blood cultures |
| **Imaging in increasing order of sensitivity and specificity** | X-ray, radionucleotide bone scanning, CT, and MRI |
| **What's the problem with x-ray?** | May not be positive until at least 10 days after infection |
| **So, if your clinical suspicion is high and the x-ray is negative, should you order additional imaging?** | Yes |

| | |
|---|---|
| **What is a common radiographic report for osteomyelitis?** | Destruction of normal bony architecture (bone erosion, periosteal elevation) with evidence of soft tissue swelling |
| **Is imaging enough for the diagnosis?** | No, it is suggestive. |
| **What additional diagnostic test should you order to support the diagnosis and direct therapy?** | Gram stain and culture of needle-aspirated pus from the bone |
| **How is the diagnosis ultimately made?** | Bone biopsy and culture of specimen |
| **What causative organisms do you suspect in** | |
| **Nondiabetic?** | *Staphylococcus aureus* and coagulase-negative staphylococci |
| **Diabetics?** | Polymicrobial infections with Gram-negative rods and anaerobes |
| **What's your empiric therapy for** | |
| **Gram-positive?** | Nafcillin |
| **Gram-negative?** | Third-generation cephalosporin (ceftriaxone) |
| **What will determine which antibiotic to continue treatment with?** | Culture and sensitivity results |
| **How long will you need to treat for?** | 4–6 weeks |
| **When is surgical debridement necessary?** | Failed medical treatment, undrained pus, or septic arthritis |

## THE SERONEGATIVE SPONDYLOARTHROPATHIES

| | |
|---|---|
| **Name the four spondyloarthropathies** | Ankylosing spondylitis, Reiter syndrome, colitic arthritis, psoriatic arthritis |

| | |
|---|---|
| **What do they have in common?** | Spondylitis, sacroilitis, inflammation at the tendon insertion points (enthesopathy), asymmetric oligoarthritis, extraarticular finding (inflammatory eye disease, urethritis, mucocutaneous lesions), and HLA-B27 association |

## CASE 9

*A 23-year-old male presents with complaints of gradual onset of morning stiffness and low back pain that worsens with rest and improves with activity.*

| | |
|---|---|
| **What's your differential diagnosis?** | Ankylosing spondylitis, Reiter syndrome, rheumatoid arthritis, musculoskeletal strain |
| **What's most likely?** | Ankylosing spondylitis |
| **Why?** | Male, under 40, morning stiffness and low back pain that lessen with activity is classic presentation |
| **What causes ankylosing spondylitis?** | Inflammation and ossification of joints and ligaments of the spine and sacroiliac joints (hips and shoulder most common) of unknown etiology |
| **What do you expect to find on physical exam?** | Decreased range of motion in lumbar spine and loss of lumbar lordosis |
| **What lab tests will you order to support your diagnosis?** | Elevated HLA-B27 and ESR and absent rheumatoid factor |
| **What diagnostic imaging study should you order?** | X-ray of the lumbar spine and sacroiliac joints |
| **What diagnostic phrase do you expect to read in the report?** | "Bamboo-spine" with fusion of the sacroiliac joints |
| **The diagnosis of ankylosing spondylitis is made. What's your treatment?** | NSAIDs (indomethacin) for symptomatic relief, physical therapy, and sleep on a firm bed without a pillow |

## CASE 10

*A 24-year-old male presents with history of diarrhea 3 weeks ago and returns to the clinic with redness in the eyes, tearing, painful urination, mouth sores, and right knee pain.*

| | |
|---|---|
| **What's your differential diagnosis?** | Reiter syndrome, arthritis associated with IBD, gonococcal arthritis, juvenile rheumatoid arthritis |
| **Which is most likely?** | Reiter syndrome |
| **What's another name for it?** | Reactive arthritis |
| **Why is it called this?** | It often occurs after (reacting to) STD or diarrhea (as in this patient) |
| **Which organisms are associated with the diarrhea seen in Reiter syndrome?** | *Salmonella, Shigella,* or *Yersinia* |
| **What classic triad of Reiter's did this patient present with?** | Conjunctivitis (redness in the eyes, tearing), urethritis (painful urination), and asymmetric oligoarthritis (right knee pain) |
| **What lab test findings do you expect?** | Positive HLA-B27, elevated WBC and ESR |
| **How will you make the diagnosis?** | Clinical history and presentation |
| **What is the treatment?** | NSAIDs (indomethacin) for pain and inflammation, referral to ophthalmologist if suspect uveitis, treat underlying STD if present |

## CASE 11

*A 22-year-old female with a long history of ulcerative colitis who has experienced a recent flare due to noncompliance with her rx medication presents with bloody diarrhea and knee and ankle pain.*

| | |
|---|---|
| **What's your brief differential diagnosis?** | Septic arthritis, colitic arthritis, gonococcal arthritis |
| **What is the most likely explanation for her joint pain?** | Ulcerative colitis (UC) flare causing colitic arthritis |
| **Why?** | History of IBD, peripheral joint discomfort (not spinal) |
| **What other extraintestinal features of IBD may be found on exam?** | Pyodermic gangrenosum, uveitis, erythema nodosum |
| **Should joint aspiration be considered?** | Yes, it will help rule out septic arthritis. |
| **What lab tests should you order?** | Stool studies, UA, HLA-B27, CBC, and blood cultures if suspect bacteremia |
| **How is the diagnosis made?** | Clinical presentation and a negative HLA-B27 lab test |
| **What is the treatment?** | Sulfasalazine for intestinal inflammation and NSAIDs for peripheral arthritis; local injection of glucocorticoids and physical therapy may be used as needed. |

## CASE 12

*A 31-year-old female with known psoriasis and IBS presents with complaints of swollen tender fingers. On exam you confirm distal interphalangea (DIP) joint swelling, warmth, tenderness, and restricted motion with pitting of the nails.*

| | |
|---|---|
| **What's your differential diagnosis?** | Psoriatic arthritis, gout, Reiter syndrome, osteoarthritis (OA) |
| **Which is most likely?** | Psoriatic arthritis |
| **Why?** | Asymmetric oligoarthritis or symmetric polyarthritis presenting in a patient with known psoriasis and nail pitting is highly suggestive of psoriatic arthritis. |

| | |
|---|---|
| **What is a classic description of the DIP joint on exams?** | Sausage shaped |
| **What radiographic image should you order?** | Hand x-ray |
| **What classic radiographic finding do you suspect?** | Pencil and cup deformity of the phalynx |
| **How will you make the diagnosis?** | Clinical presentation with associated psoriatic findings on the skin, nail, and hair |
| **How is it distinguished from rhematoid arthritis?** | Rheumatoid factor is negative in psoriatic arthritis |
| **What is the treatment?** | NSAIDs (indomethacin), intraarticular steroids if oligoarticular form of the disease |

## OSTEOARTHRITIS AND ARTHROPATHIES

### CASE 13

*A 37-year-old previously healthy male presents with difficulty walking due to severe pain, swelling, redness, and warmth of his right great toe over the last 24 hours after partying all night at a friend's bachelor party. His hangover has subsided, but his big toe pain continues despite taking Tylenol.*

| | |
|---|---|
| **What's your differential diagnosis?** | Gout, pseudogout, hyperparathyroidism, fracture secondary to trauma sustained while intoxicated |
| **Which is most likely?** | Gout |
| **Why?** | Acute attack of excruciating pain in a single joint of the foot or ankle, most commonly the big toe (Podagra), is classic for gout. |
| **What could have triggered this attack?** | Dehydration and high alcohol intake |

| | |
|---|---|
| **What other risk factors for gout are there?** | Surgery, fasting, and binge eating (meat) |
| **What lab tests should you order?** | CBC, ESR, and serum uric acid |
| **Is hyperuricemia required to make the diagnosis?** | No, one-third of patients have normal serum uric acid levels during an acute attack. |
| **How will you make the diagnosis?** | Aspirate the joint |
| **What finding is diagnostic?** | Needle-shaped negatively birefringent crystals within PMNs under a polarized light microscope |
| **What causes gout?** | An inborn error in uric acid metabolism leads to crystal deposition in the peripheral joints. |
| **What is the first line of treatment?** | High-dose oral NSAIDs or colchicine (if contraindication to NSAID use) |
| **Name two common contraindications to NSAID use.** | History of NSAID-related bleed and advanced renal insufficiency |
| **What prophylactic medications can be used between attacks?** | Allopurinol 300 mg daily (if consistent hyperuricemia due to uric acid overproduction) or probenecid (if chronic underexcretion of uric acid = less than 700 mg in urine per 24 hours) |

## CASE 14

*A 55-year-old obese male with history of HTN, diabetes, and lumbago presents with bilateral knee pain that has worsened slowly over the last 2 years. The knee pain is worse in the morning, lasts less than 30 minutes, and improves with activity.*

| | |
|---|---|
| **What diagnosis do you suspect?** | Osteoarthritis (OA, also known as degenerative joint disease) |

**What causes OA?**

Deterioration of the articular cartilage and formation of reactive new bone at the articular surface in one or more joints

**What in the history is consistent with OA?**

**Age**

Most often over 40 (he's 55)

**Weight**

Obesity

**Joints affected**

Those under chronic use or weight bearing

**Symptom onset and duration**

Short-lived morning stiffness and pain (often less than 30 minutes)

**What do you expect to find on physical exam?**

Decreased range of joint motion, pain with movement, small effusions, and crepitus

**What physical exam finding would be present in patients with OA in the hands from overuse?**

Heberdon nodes (body deformity at DIP common) and Bouchard nodes (bony deformity at PIP less common)

**Are blood tests required to make the diagnosis?**

No, patients have normal WBC and ESR.

**What would be found if the joint was aspirated?**

Straw-colored joint fluid with few WBCs

**What imaging should be ordered?**

Plain-x-rays of affected joints

**What findings do you expect?**

Joint space narrowing with osteophytes

**How is it diagnosed?**

Clinical exam and x-ray findings

**What's your first line of therapy?**

NSAIDs or aspirin, weight reduction, exercise, physical therapy

**What if these fail and the patient is severely disabled?**

Total joint replacement (knee replacement most common)

CASE 15

*A 68-year-old male with history of hemochromatosis, diabetes, and hypertension presents with left knee warmth and tenderness that has progressed over the last week.*

| | |
|---|---|
| **What's your differential diagnosis?** | Gout, pseudogout, septic arthritis, or trauma |
| **What tests should you order?** | |
| Labs | CBC, ESR, PT, and INR |
| Imaging | X-ray |
| Procedure | Aspiration of knee synovial fluid |
| **How will you make the diagnosis?** | Synovial fluid analysis |
| **Synovial fluid analyzed under polarized light microscope shows positively birefringent rhomboid-shaped crystals. What's your diagnosis?** | Pseudogout |
| **What causes pseudogout?** | Accumulation of calcium pyrophosphate crystals in the peripheral joint space |
| **What risk factors did this patient have for pseudogout?** | Old age, hemochromatosis, and diabetes |
| **Name other risk factors.** | Trauma, advanced osteoarthritis, gout, hyperparathyroidism, hypothyroidism, and amyloidosis |
| **What joint is most commonly affected?** | Knee (as in this patient) |
| **What is the treatment?** | Brief high-dose course of NSAIDs (indomethacin) |

## CASE 16

*A 33-year-old female with history of UTIs presents with morning stiffness last-
ing 90 minutes with fatigue, weakness, and tender knuckles. On exam you
find symmetrical PIP and MCP tenderness and swelling.*

| | |
|---|---|
| **What's your differential diagnosis?** | Rheumatoid arthritis, gout, erosive osteoarthritis, pseudogout, SLE |
| **Which is most likely?** | Rheumatoid arthritis (RA) |
| **What supports RA?** | |
| Age | Often presents in second to fifth decade (she's 33) |
| **Gender** | Females > Males |
| **Common symptoms** | Significant morning stiffness lasting more than 1 hour with fatigue, weakness, and joint pain |
| **Physical exam findings** | Symmetrical joint pain, tenderness, swelling, and warmth that most commonly involves the hands (PIP and MCP joints very common, DIP spared) |
| **What other joints can be affected?** | Wrists, elbows, ankles, and feet |
| **What tests should you order?** | CBC, ESR, RF, synovial fluid analysis |
| **What results would support RA in the** | |
| CBC? | Mild anemia |
| ESR? | Elevated |
| RF? | >1:80 |
| Synovial fluid? | Yellow-white, turbid fluid with WBC in the range of 3500–50,000 |

| | |
|---|---|
| **How is the diagnosis made?** | A positive rheumatoid factor with an elevated sedimentation rate with presentation of significant morning stiffness lasting more than 1 hour and symmetric polyarthritis |
| **What causes RA?** | A chronic systemic inflammatory disease of unknown etiology causing symmetric joint inflammation, deformation, and bone erosion from chronic synovial inflammation |
| **Describe 2 syndromes associated with RA** | Felty Syndrome (RA, splenomegaly grand ocynpenia) Sjögren Syndrome (dry eyes, mouth, parotid gland enlargement) |
| **What is the treatment for mild to moderate cases?** | NSAIDs to reduce pain and swelling and disease-modifying drugs like methotrexate or hydroxychloroquine |
| **What medications are considered for moderate to severe cases or those unresponsive to first-line therapy?** | Short-term steroid use or TNF inhibitor medications like enterecept (Enbrel) or infliximab (Remicade) |
| **What additional non-medical treatment may be helpful?** | Physical therapy |
| **When is surgery warranted?** | When other therapies have failed to reduce chronic pain and improve joint function |

## CASE 17

*A 19-year-old female presents to the ER with her mother complaining of right knee pain with difficulty bending it. She plays soccer and has injured her knee before and twisted it last week during practice, but is concerned because it is not getting better. On exam the right knee is tender, warm, erythematous, and swollen with minor superficial abrasions.*

**What's your differential diagnosis?**

Gout, pseudogout, septic arthritis, spondyloarthropathy, juvenile rheumatoid arthritis, foreign body synovitis, rheumatoid arthritis, rheumatic fever, AIDS, cellulites, lyme arthritis, neuropathic arthropathy, and sarcoidosis

**What risk factor does she have for septic arthritis stated in the history?**

Trauma (although minor and unlikely the culprit)

**What additional history should you obtain?**

Sexual history and IVDA abuse, after excusing mother from the room

**Why? What are you considering?**

Septic arthritis possibly secondary to gonococcus or staphylococcus

**Which joint is commonly involved in both?**

Large joints (knee or hip most commonly)

**What in the history is inconsistent with gonococcal septic arthritis?**

Gonococcal cases often begin as a migratory polyarthralgia that becomes a monoarthritis, tenosynovitis of the wrists, fingers, knees, and ankles, a maculopapular or vesicular dermatitis of the lower extremities or trunk, all of which are absent in her presentation.

**What's your diagnostic approach?**

Aspirate joint fluid for WBC count, culture, and Gram stain; blood cultures; all orifices cultured for gonorrhea in Thayer-Martin medium

**When gonorrhea is under consideration, what additional test should be ordered?**

Syphilis serology

**What's your most important diagnostic test?**

Aspirate synovial fluid from the joint

**The synovial fluid is turbid, WBC count of 78,000 cell/μL, and PMNs of 92%. What's your diagnosis?**

Septic arthritis

**What is the diagnostic criteria for septic arthritis?**

Turbid fluid, WBC count greater than 50,000 cells/μL, PMNs greater than 90%

**What's your initial treatment?**

(1) Hospitalize for intravenous antibiotics

(2) Immobilize the joint

**What dictates antibiotic selection?**

Gram stain and culture results

**The culture is positive for staphylococci. What is your treatment?**

Intravenous nafcillin or vancomycin followed by an oral antibiotic (dicloxacillin) for a total of 3–6 weeks

**What if the Gram stain was positive for gonococci?**

Ceftriaxone 1 g daily for 14 days (but at least 7 days after symptoms resolve)

**When should surgery be consulted with septic joints?**

Septic hip, inadequate needle drainage, no response to therapy after 5–7 days, coexistent osteomyelitis, or prosthetic joint infection, none of which is present in this patient

# 9     Dermatology

## SKIN ERUPTIONS

### CASE 1

*A 14-year-old girl is distraught because her face has broken out with skin lesions (Figures 9-1 and 9-2). On examination you confirm that the skin condition is limited to the face.*

| | |
|---|---|
| **Describe the lesions.** | Papular lesion with open (whitehead) and closed (blackhead) comedomes |
| **What's your most likely diagnosis?** | Mild facial acne |
| **What's the differential diagnosis for facial acne?** | *Staphylococcus aureus* folliculitis, pseudofolliculitis barbae, rosacea, and periorbital dermatitis |
| **Why is acne most likely in the differential diagnosis?** | Because it is the most common facial skin condition presenting in adolescents (especially at puberty) |
| **How is acne diagnosed?** | History and physical exam |

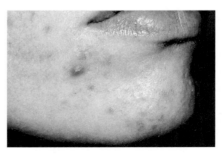

**Figure 9–1.**
*Source:* Goodheart HP. Goodheart's Photoguide of Common Skin Disorders, 2nd Ed. Philadelphia: Lippincott Williams & Wilkins, 2003.

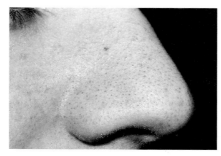

**Figure 9–2.**
*Source:* Goodheart HP. Goodheart's Photoguide of Common Skin Disorders, 2nd Ed. Philadelphia: Lippincott Williams & Wilkins, 2003.

| | |
|---|---|
| **What causes it?** | A multifactorial process associated with excess sebum production, overgrowth of *Propionibacterium acnes,* androgen excess, inflammation, and abnormal keratin production causing hair follicle plugging |
| **What treatments are available?** | Benzoyl peroxide (decreases *P. acne*), retinoic acid (decreases abnormal keratin production), and topical antibiotics (erythromycin and clindamycin) |

## CASE 2

A 65-year-old avid golfer living in Florida with a history of ulcerative colitis on a small dose of prednisone and immuran (steroid sparring agent) presents with well-marginated, reddish papule with rough (feels like sandpaper) yellow-brown scales < 1 cm on sun-exposed skin (Figure 9-3).

| | |
|---|---|
| **What is your differential diagnosis?** | SCC, flat warts, superficial BCC, aktinic keratosis |
| **Which is most likely?** | Actinic keratosis (AK) |
| **Why?** | His frequently sun-exposed skin (golf) and immunocompromised status (on immuran) are strong risk factors for AK. |

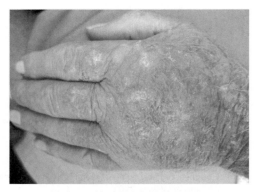

**Figure 9–3.** Image provided by Stedman's.

| | |
|---|---|
| **Is clinical history and PE enough to make the diagnosis?** | No, you must perform a skin biopsy to exclude cancer. |
| **The biopsy confirms AK; what did the pathologist see?** | Clonal proliferation of atypical keratinocytes |
| **Why is it important to treat AK?** | Untreated patients are at risk for SCC (1:1000 risk). |
| **What is the treatment?** | Cryosurgery (preferred), topical 5-fluorouracil cream, or electrocautery |

## CASE 3

*A morbidly obese woman with uncontrolled diabetes and chronic obstructive pulmonary disease (COPD) on steroid inhalers presents with itching and burning sensation in the inner thighs and pain with swallowing. On exam you find beefy-red lesions of varying sizes on warm moist areas of the body (inner thigh, axillae, beneath breasts) (Figure 9-4) and white plaques on the tongue (Figure 9-5).*

| | |
|---|---|
| **What do you see?** | Small peripheral papules and pustules that have become confluent centrally giving a beefy-red appearance |

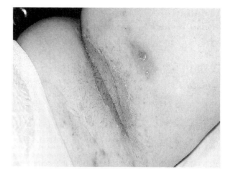

**Figure 9–4.**
*Source:* Goodheart HP. Goodheart's Photoguide of Common Skin Disorders, 2nd Ed. Philadelphia: Lippincott Williams & Wilkins, 2003.

**What's your differential diagnosis?**

Cutaneous candidiasis, impetigo, eczematous dermatitis, psoriasis, dermatophytosis, pityriasis versicolor

**What do you see?**

White plagues on the oral mucosa and tongue

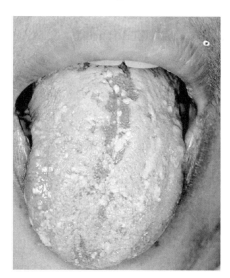

**Figure 9–5.**
*Source:* Goodheart HP. Goodheart's Photoguide of Common Skin Disorders, 2nd Ed. Philadelphia: Lippincott Williams & Wilkins, 2003.

| | |
|---|---|
| **What's your differential diagnosis for the oral lesion?** | Oral candidiasis, hairy leukoplaki, hyperkeratosis, lichen planus, squamous cell carcinoma (SCC) |
| **What organism could be causing both of these lesions?** | *Candida albicans* |
| **How do you make the diagnosis?** | Microscopic visualization of yeast and pseudohyphae using 10% potassium hydroxide |
| **What risk factors did this patient have to develop candidiasis?** | Diabetic, obesity, and steroid inhaler (probably swallowed and failed to rinse mouth out after use) |
| **What additional risk factor needs to be considered when oral candidiasis presents?** | Immunosuppression (HIV/AIDS?) |
| **What is the treatment for** | |
|    **Skin lesions?** | Nystatin cream and ketoconazole cream |
|    **Oral candidiasis?** | Nystatin liquid ("swish and swallow") |

## CASE 4

*A 68-year-old woman with uncontrolled diabetes with end-stage manifestations of neuropathy, vascular insufficiency, and retinopathy presents with pain in left ankle after tripping over a vacuum cleaner last week. On exam you find a small ulcer that's tender, warm, and red with a diffuse border (Figure 9-6).*

| | |
|---|---|
| **How would you describe this?** | Small, shallow ulcer with peripheral erythema, edema, and diffuse border |
| **What most likely caused it?** | A polymicrobial bacterial infection secondary to skin trauma (tripped over vacuum cleaner) in a patient with vascular insufficiency secondary to diabetes mellitis |
| **What risk factors does this patient have?** | Diabetes, skin trauma, vascular insufficiency |

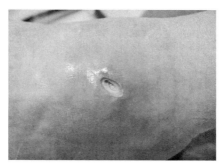

**Figure 9–6.** Image provided by Stedman's.

| | |
|---|---|
| **What other risk factors exist?** | Immunosuppression, lymphatic and venous obstruction |
| **What labs should you order?** | CBC, Gram stain and cultures of skin lesions, blood cultures, and possible skin biopsy |
| **What empiric antibiotics should you prescribe after cultures are obtained?** | Oxacillin or a cephazolin |
| **What organisms are you targeting?** | Group A β-hemolytic streptococci and *Staphylococcus aureus* |
| **What additional treatment may be required in diabetics?** | Anaerobic antibiotics (e.g., metronidazole or clindamycin) because of increased risk of polymicrobial infection |

CASE 5

A 48-year-old female comes to the emergency room after wearing latex gloves for the first time with new onset of bilateral hand redness, pruritis, and swelling (Figure 9-7).

| | |
|---|---|
| **What is the most likely cause?** | Mild contact dermatitis from a latex allergy |
| **How would a severe case present?** | Severe swelling and blistering |

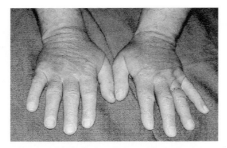

**Figure 9–7.**
*Source:* Goodheart HP. Goodheart's Photoguide of Common Skin Disorders, 2nd Ed.
Philadelphia: Lippincott Williams & Wilkins, 2003.

| | |
|---|---|
| **What other common causes of contact dermatitis are there?** | Soaps, detergents, dyes, solvents, drugs, cosmetics, poison ivy, poison oak, rubber, latex, metals |
| **How is contact dermatitis diagnosed?** | History and patch testing |
| **What is the treatment?** | Remove and avoid irritant, wash affected area with soap and water, antihistamine (pruritis), and topical corticosteroids |
| **What therapy modification is made in severe cases (especially if face is affected)?** | Systemic steroids (prednisone) |

## CASE 6

*A 77-year-old woman with history of HTN, stressed out over her son's wedding, developed low grade fever, malaise, and a tingling pain in her abdomen beginning around the umbilicus and radiating around to the back.*

| | |
|---|---|
| **What's your differential diagnosis?** | Herpes zoster, cholecystitis, pleuritis, acute abdomen, diabetic neuropathy, vertebral radicular disease |
| **Your physical exam and lab results are normal. What's your most likely diagnosis?** | Herpes zoster ("shingles") |

**Why?**

Prodrome symptoms in a patient with pain in a dermatomal distribution with normal PE and labs

**When will the rash appear?**

3 days from onset of prodrome symptoms

**Describe the rash that will develop.**

Erythematous and maculopapular rash that rapidly progresses to grouped vesicles that become pustular and crust over; hemorrhagic crusts may be present (Figure 9-8)

**What is the differential diagnosis when a patient presents with a shingles-like rash?**

Herpes simplex virus, poison ivy or poison oak, contact dermatitis

**What was this patient's risk factor?**

Elderly

**What other risk factors should be considered?**

Immunocompromised (unlikely in this patient), spinal surgery, spinal cord radiation

**How is the diagnosis often made?**

History and presentation

**What test would confirm the diagnosis?**

Positive Tzanck smear demonstrating multinucleated giant cells

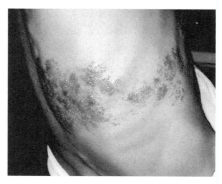

**Figure 9–8.**
*Source:* Goodheart HP. Goodheart's Photoguide of Common Skin Disorders, 2nd Ed. Philadelphia: Lippincott Williams & Wilkins, 2003.

| | |
|---|---|
| **What is the problem with the Tzanck smear?** | It is also positive for herpes simplex virus and a false-negative may occur |
| **What causes shingles?** | A latent reaction to the varicella-zoster virus from a prior chicken pox (herpes varicella) infection |
| **Where was the virus hiding?** | Sensory nerve ganglia |
| **What is the treatment?** | Analgesics, topical calamine lotion, contact isolation precautions while rash is present (it is contagious) |
| **What additional treatment is used in immunocompromised patients?** | Acyclovir |

CASE 7

_A 23-year-old man presents with silvery scales on bright red, well-demarcated plaques most often on the knees, elbows, and scalp (Figure 9-9)._

| | |
|---|---|
| **What's your differential diagnosis?** | Psoriasis, seborrheic dermatitis, lichen simplex chronicus, candidiasis, psoriasiform drug eruption, tinea corporus, mycosis fungoides |
| **What is your most likely diagnosis?** | Psoriasis |
| **Why?** | Distribution of rash on knees, elbows, and scalp is classic for psoriasis. |

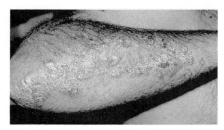

**Figure 9–9.**
_Source:_ Goodheart HP. Goodheart's Photoguide of Common Skin Disorders, 2nd Ed. Philadelphia: Lippincott Williams & Wilkins, 2003.

| | |
|---|---|
| **Is family history important?** | Yes, because the risk of developing the rash is significantly increased if present in the parents. |
| **What additional finding on physical exam would support psoriasis?** | Nail pitting or onycholysis |
| **How is the diagnosis made?** | History and presentation |
| **What confirms the diagnosis?** | Skin biopsy (although often not required) |
| **What are some of the pathologic findings in psoriasis?** | Marked epidermal thickening, increased mitosis of keratinocytes, and inflammatory cells in the dermis |
| **What is the basic problem in this disease?** | Keratinocytes produce roughly 28 times the normal quantity of epidermal cells. |
| **What treatments are available?** | Ultraviolet light, topical corticosteroids, and topical tar |

## CASE 8

An 8-year-old boy presents with intense itching in the finger web spaces and flexor surfaces of the wrists. On physical exam the linear tan ridges are identified with small vesicles or papules at the end (Figure 9-10).

| | |
|---|---|
| **What's your differential diagnosis?** | Scabies, drug reaction, contact dermatitis |
| **Which is most likely?** | Scabies |
| **Why?** | Scabies commonly presents with intensely pruritic erythematous papular skin lesions. |
| **What are common sites for scabies infection?** | Hands (often flexor surfaces), axillary folds, trunk, buttocks, and genitalia |
| **How long are lesions typically?** | 2–3 mm long and the width of a hair |

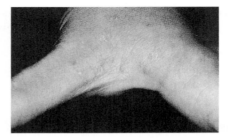

**Figure 9–10.**
*Source:* Fleisher GR, Ludwig S, Baskin MN. Atlas of Pediatric Emergency Medicine.
Philadelphia: Lippincott Williams & Wilkins, 2004.

| | |
|---|---|
| **How will you make the diagnosis?** | Scrape the lesion and look for the scabies mite, eggs, or feces under the microscope |
| **What causes scabies?** | Female sarcoptes scabiei ("itch mite") lay eggs in the skin that release larvae that irritate the hair follicles |
| **What is the treatment?** | Permethrin 5% cream (preferred) or lindane 1% cream (neurotoxicity risk). Wash all clothing, sheets, and linens in hot water. |

## CASE 9

*A 19-year-old male with history of drug abuse and multiple sexual partners over the last year presents with a painless ulcer pictured (Figure 9-11).*

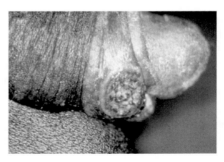

**Figure 9–11.**
*Source:* Goodheart HP. Goodheart's Photoguide of Common Skin Disorders, 2nd Ed.
Philadelphia: Lippincott Williams & Wilkins, 2003.

| | |
|---|---|
| **What is your differential diagnosis?** | Primary syphilis, chancroid, lymphogranuloma venereum, granuloma inguinale, herpes, Beschet syndrome, trauma |
| **Your physical exam confirms as pictured above. What is the most likely diagnosis?** | Primary syphilis |
| **Why?** | A painless, indurated, superficial ulceration in a patient with multiple sexual partners is consistent with syphilis. |
| **What are the risk factors for contracting syphilis?** | Sexual contact (most common and most likely in this patient), blood transfusions, and vertical transmission from mother to infant |
| **When was he most likely exposed?** | 3 weeks ago (typical incubation period) |
| **What diagnostic tests are available?** | |
| **Inexpensive serologic** | Venereal disease research laboratory and rapid plasma regain |
| **Expensive serologic** | Fluorescent treponemal antibody absorption test and microhemagglutinin antigen-treponeum pallidum |
| **Microscopy** | Dark-field microscopy of lesion exudates to reveal the spirochete *Treponema pallidum* |
| **How is diagnosis made?** | History, presentation, and positive serologic studies or microscopy |
| **What is the treatment?** | Benzathine penicillin G, 2.4 million units in a single dose |
| **If the patient refuses therapy, how long will it take the chancre to heal?** | 6–8 weeks |

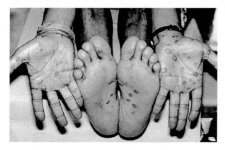

**Figure 9–12.**
*Source:* Goodheart HP. Goodheart's Photoguide of Common Skin Disorders, 2nd Ed.
Philadelphia: Lippincott Williams & Wilkins, 2003.

| | |
|---|---|
| **What can occur if primary syphilis is not treated?** | Secondary or tertiary syphilis |
| **Give examples of possible presentations for both.** | |
| **Secondary syphilis** | Flu-like illness (malaise, headache, anorexia), generalized nontender lymphadenopathy, and a maculopapular rash [especially on palms and soles as shown (Figure 9-12)]. |
| **Tertiary syphilis** | Cutaneous gumma, aortic aneurysms, general paresis, tabes dorsalis, or meningitis |

## CASE 10

*A 55-year-old retired professional caddy for Jack Nicklaus presents with a rash on his nose that has failed therapy with self-prescribed over-the-counter medication (Figure 9-13).*

| | |
|---|---|
| **What's your differential diagnosis?** | Basal cell carcinoma (BCC), sebaceous hyperplasia, intradermal nevi, molluscum contagiosum |
| **What is most likely?** | BCC |

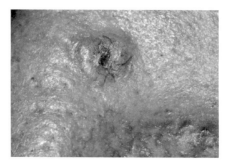

**Figure 9–13.**
*Source:* Goodheart HP. Goodheart's Photoguide of Common Skin Disorders, 2nd Ed. Philadelphia: Lippincott Williams & Wilkins, 2003.

| | |
|---|---|
| **Why?** | Classic risk factors of excessive exposure to sunlight (professional caddy), light-skinned person (Irish) with presentation on sun-exposed area is highly suspicious for BCC. |
| **What is the natural history of the BCC lesion?** | Begins as a pale, "pearly" papule with dilated blood vessels (telangiectasia) that enlarges peripherally and develops a central depression or ulceration that crusts and bleeds |
| **How do you make the diagnosis?** | Biopsy |
| **What would be seen by the pathologist?** | A nidus of epidermal basal cells extending into the dermis with large basophilic oval nuclei |
| **What's the treatment?** | Surgical excision |

CASE 11

*A 45-year-old woman with history of noninsulin-dependent diabetes and a severe sunburn as a child presents with a dark spot on her skin (Figure 9-14).*

| | |
|---|---|
| **What's your differential diagnosis?** | Malignant melanoma, dysplastic nevi, vascular skin tumors, BCC |
| **Which is most likely?** | Malignant melanoma |

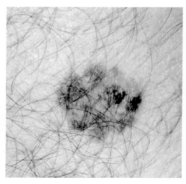

**Figure 9–14.**
*Source:* Goodheart HP. Goodheart's Photoguide of Common Skin Disorders, 2nd Ed. Philadelphia: Lippincott Williams & Wilkins, 2003.

| | |
|---|---|
| **Why?** | The pigmented lesion has the classic ABCD of melanoma: A, asymmetry; B, border irregularity; C, color variation; D, diameter >6 mm. |
| **Where is this lesion most likely found?** | Lower extremity (more common in women) |
| **What if the patient had been a man?** | Trunk |
| **Can melanoma present elsewhere?** | Yes |
| **What put this patient at risk?** | Sun exposure (severe burn in childhood) |
| **What other risk factors exist for melanoma?** | Dysplastic nevi, prior melanoma, family history (first-degree relative) and xeroderma pigmentosum |
| **How is it diagnosed?** | Excisional biopsy |
| **What will the pathology report most likely find?** | Superficial spreading melanocytes which is the most common form (70%) of melanoma |
| **What is the treatment?** | Wide excision |

## CASE 12

*A 62-year-old fair-skinned male golf course greens-keeper with history of diabetes and actinic keratosis presents with a new skin lesion (Figure 9-15).*

**What is your differential diagnosis?**

Squamous cell carcinoma (SCC), BCC, aktinic keratosis, malignant melanoma, keratoacanthoma

**You are informed that it began as a crusted red papule that became nodular (and occasionally ulcerates). What is your most likely diagnosis?**

SCC

**What are this patient's risk factors for SCC?**

Older age (up to ten times risk in elderly), male (2–3 × risk), sun exposure (greens-keeper), fair skin, actinic keratosis

**How will you confirm your diagnosis of SCC?**

Skin biopsy

**What will the pathology report say?**

Atypical epithelial cells arising from the epidermis and extending into the dermis consistent with SCC

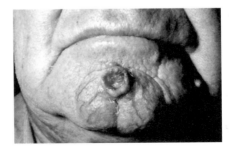

**Figure 9–15.**
*Source:* Weber J, Kelley J. Health Assessment in Nursing, 2nd Ed. Philadelphia: Lippincott Williams & Wilkins, 2003.

| **What specific epithelial cell does SCC arise from?** | Keratinocytes |

| **What is the treatment?** | Surgical excision |

## CASE 13

A 16-year-old boy presents with a painless, firm, well-circumscribed nodule with cornified epithelium (Figure 9-16).

| **What is your differential diagnosis?** | Viral wart, scar tissue, molluscum contagiosum, condyloma lata, seborrheic keratosis |
| **Which diagnosis do you suspect?** | Viral warts (verruca vulgaris) |
| **Where do viral warts commonly appear?** | Fingers, knees, elbows, and feet |
| **What size are they?** | Less than 1 cm |
| **What are the risk factors to ask about?** | Local irritation, trauma, immunosuppressive diseases or drug use, atopic dermatitis |
| **How is the diagnosis often made?** | Clinically |

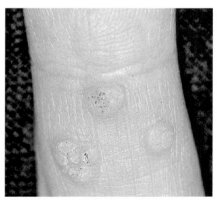

**Figure 9–16.**
*Source:* Goodheart HP. Goodheart's Photoguide of Common Skin Disorders, 2nd Ed. Philadelphia: Lippincott Williams & Wilkins, 2003.

| How would you confirm it? | Biopsy |
| --- | --- |
| **What would the pathology report say?** | Human papilloma virus (HPV) found in the nuclei and nucleoli of the epidermal stratum granulosum and keratin layers |
| **What is the treatment?** | Topical salicylic acid or cryotherapy |

## CASE 14

*An 18-year-old African American male presents after having sutures removed 3 weeks ago for a laceration during a motor vehicle accident with an enlarging well-demarcated scar (Figure 9-17).*

| **What's your differential diagnosis?** | Keloid, hypertropic scar, dermatofibroma, BCC |
| --- | --- |
| **Which is most likely?** | Keloid |
| **Why?** | Patient has classic risk factors and presentation for keloid formation |
| **What are his risk factors?** | Dark skin pigment (African American), adolescence, and recent skin trauma in same location |

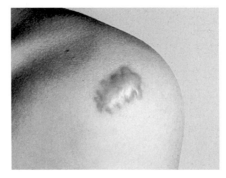

**Figure 9–17.**
*Source:* Willis MC. Medical Terminology: A Programmed Learning Approach to the Language of Health Care. Baltimore: Lippincott Williams & Wilkins, 2002.

| | |
|---|---|
| **What are other risk factors for keloid formation?** | Pregnancy, inflammation, and family history |
| **How is the diagnosis often made?** | Clinically |
| **How could it be confirmed?** | Biopsy |
| **What would the pathology report show?** | Whorls of hyalinized collagen bundles with thinning of the dermis and decreased elastic tissue |
| **What causes it?** | Irregular organization of fibroblasts following skin injury |
| **What is the treatment?** | Local steroid injections |

## UTERUS

### CASE 1

*A 35-year-old obese African American female presents with menorrhagia for the last 4 months and a sense of pressure in the pelvis. On physical examination, you appreciate an enlarged, mobile uterus with an irregular contour on bimanual examination.*

| | |
|---|---|
| **What's your broad differential diagnosis for menorrhagia in this patient?** | Coagulopathy, structural lesion like uterine or cervical cancer, fibroids, endometriosis |
| **Which is suggested by the physical exam findings?** | Fibroids (a.k.a. leiomyoma) |
| **How do fibroids present?** | Often asymptomatic, but may present with abnormal uterine bleeding, a pelvic mass, and sensations of pressure in the pelvis |
| **What is it?** | Benign hormonally responsive uterine tumor also known as a myoma or fibroma that is composed of smooth muscle tissue which usually regresses after menopause |
| **What are this patient's risk factors?** | African American and obesity |
| **What other risk factors have been reported?** | Premenopausal, nonsmokers |
| **Describe findings on the following tests that support the diagnosis of fibroids:** | |
| Physical exam | Enlarged, mobile uterus with an irregular contour on bimanual examination |
| Abdominal x-ray | Discrete, calcified round masses |

| | |
|---|---|
| **Hysterosalpingography** | Distinct areas lacking contrast |
| **Ultrasound** | "Snowstorm" image |
| **What additional procedure is required if the diagnosis is uncertain?** | Biopsy of suspicious mass |

**What is the treatment strategy in**

| | |
|---|---|
| **Asymptomatic patients?** | None as the fibroids shrink after menopause |
| **Symptomatic patients?** | Gonadotropin-releasing hormone agonists result in decreased LH and FSH with resultant menopause-like state |
| **What are the indications for surgery?** | A rapidly growing myoma in a menopausal female usually warrants hysterectomy or myomectomy. |

## CASE 2

*A 31-year-old female G0P0 presents to your clinic with her husband after being unable to get pregnant after trying for 6 months. She also complains of abnormal menstrual bleeding and worsening pain with menses.*

| | |
|---|---|
| **What is the differential diagnosis?** | Pelvic inflammatory disease (PID), ovarian cancer, and leiomyomas |
| **Which is most likely?** | Endometriosis |
| **What were the clues?** | Progressive dysmenorrhea, dyspareunia, abnormal bleeding, cyclical pelvic pain, and infertility are suggestive of endometriosis. |
| **What is endometriosis?** | Ectopic growth of uterine glands and stroma |
| **What are the most common locations?** | Ovary and pelvic peritoneum |
| **Name the main risk factor.** | Family history |

| | |
|---|---|
| **What may be appreciated on physical exam?** | Uterosacral nodularity on rectovaginal examination or a fixed retroverted uterus |
| **What labs should be included in the workup?** | CBC and ESR (may suggest an acute or chronic inflammatory process), UA and urine culture to rule out urologic source (e.g., cystitis, stones), and a pregnancy test and tests for sexually transmitted diseases (gonorrhea, chlamydia), when appropriate |
| **What imaging is useful?** | Abdominal ultrasound |
| **What's the definitive diagnostic test?** | Laparoscopy |
| **What's the medical treatment?** | Danzol, GnRH analogs, and estrogen-progesterone oral contraceptives |
| **What alternative therapy is available if medical therapy fails?** | Laparoscopic excision |
| **What definitive therapy exists?** | Total abdominal hysterectomy and bilateral salpingo-oophorectomy (TAHBSO) |

## CASE 3

*A 55-year-old postmenopausal women presents to your clinic complaining of vaginal bleeding for the last 6 weeks.*

| | |
|---|---|
| **What are you most concerned about?** | Endometrial cancer |
| **Why?** | Abnormal vaginal bleeding (especially in postmenopausal women) is the most common presentation. |
| **What causes it?** | Chronic exposure to unopposed estrogen |
| **What are the risk factors?** | Exogenous estrogen use, obesity, nulliparity, early menarche, late menopause, anovulatory cycles, diabetes mellitus, and polycystic ovarian syndrome |

| | |
|---|---|
| **What's in your differential diagnosis?** | Endometrial atrophy, polyp, hyperplasia, hormonal effect, and cervical cancer |
| **What tests are included in the workup?** | Speculum exam, pap smear, and endometrial biopsy |
| **How is endometrial cancer diagnosed?** | Endometrial biopsy |
| **What is the most common histologic type?** | Adenocarcinoma |
| **What radiologic test is useful to screen for metastasis?** | Chest x-ray |
| **What is the treatment for stage 1 cancer (confined to endometrium)?** | TAHBSO |
| **What additional therapy is available for more advanced disease?** | Radiation, chemotherapy, and hormone therapy (high-dose progestins and anti-estrogens) |

## OVARY

### CASE 4

*A 44-year-old G1P1 female with no known cardiac or liver disease presents to your clinic complaining of vague abdominal discomfort, increased abdominal girth, and weight loss. On exam, you appreciate abdominal distention and a fluid wave suggestive of underlying ascites.*

| | |
|---|---|
| **What's the most likely diagnosis?** | Ovarian cancer |
| **How does it present?** | Asymptomatic early on, but later vague gastrointestinal symptoms, abdominal discomfort, fullness, early satiety, ascites, pain, pelvic mass, and weight loss are common |
| **What are her risk factors?** | Middle-age and low parity |

| | |
|---|---|
| **What other risk factors should be investigated?** | Family history, delayed childbearing (over 30), and infertility |
| **What's in the differential diagnosis of ovarian cancer?** | Endometriomas, ovarian cysts, tuboovarian abscess, nongynecologic causes of a pelvic mass (e.g., colon cancer), ectopic pregnancy |
| **What must not be overlooked on the physical exam?** | Pelvic examination |
| **What physical exam findings are suggestive of ovarian cancer?** | Fixed, irregular pelvic mass with upper abdominal mass or ascites |
| **What 2 tests must be included in the workup?** | Abdominal or transvaginal ultrasound and CA-125 |
| **Why should the CA-125 be ordered?** | It is often elevated in ovarian cancer |
| **Is this tumor marker useful for screening?** | No, it is most useful to evaluate response to treatment, but is still commonly ordered on initial workup. |
| **How is the diagnosis confirmed?** | Laparotomy |
| **What's the treatment for Young patients with low-grade disease?** | Unilateral oophorectomy |
| **Advanced cases?** | Radical surgery (TAHBSO, omentectomy, debulking), radiation, and chemotherapy |

## CERVIX

CASE 5

*A 31-year-old female previously treated for human papilloma virus (HPV) presents to your clinic after having vaginal bleeding after intercourse.*

| | |
|---|---|
| **What's your most likely diagnosis?** | Cervical cancer |
| **How does it present?** | Often asymptomatic, but postcoital bleeding, abnormal vaginal bleeding, pelvic pain, and urinary tract infections may occur |
| **What known risk factor does she have?** | HPV infection |
| **What HPV types can cause it?** | HPV types 16, 18, and 31 |
| **What other risk factors should be considered?** | Cervical dysplasia, multiple sexual partners, having intercourse at an early age, and smoking |
| **What screening test should be performed?** | Pap smear |
| **How is the diagnosis confirmed?** | Biopsy |
| **What is the most common histologic type?** | Squamous cell carcinoma (about 90%) |
| **What's the treatment?** | Hysterectomy and pelvic node dissection |
| **What additional therapy is useful in advanced disease?** | Radiation and chemotherapy |

## MENSTRUAL DISORDERS

### CASE 6

*A 35-year-old female is referred to you after an extensive workup for irregular bleeding with anovulation. Her β-hCG was negative, abdominal and transvaginal ultrasound revealed normal anatomy, and serology was negative for a coagulopathy. Her pap smear and pelvic exam were unremarkable.*

| | |
|---|---|
| **What has been ruled out?** | Pregnancy, structural pelvic pathology (e.g., fibroids, polyps, etc.), cervical cancer, and coagulopathy |

| | |
|---|---|
| **What should be considered now?** | Dysfunctional uterine bleeding |
| **What is it?** | Abnormal uterine bleeding, often with anovulation, in the absence of other anatomic lesions |
| **What causes it?** | Dysfunction of the hypothalamic-pituitary-gonadal axis resulting in continuous non-cyclic estrogen stimulation of the endometrium causing it to outgrow its blood supply and slough off at irregular times and unpredictable amounts |
| **How does it often present?** | Irregular, often heavy uterine bleeding with anovulation |
| **What basic tests can be ordered to determine whether ovulation is occurring?** | A daily basal body temperature graph and day 23–35 serum progesterone level |
| **What is the gold standard test to diagnose anovulation and dysfunctional uterine bleeding?** | Endometrial biopsy |
| **What is the treatment?** | Progestational agent (e.g., medroxyprogesterone) for a minimum of 10 days during the luteal phase for several cycles |
| **What is an alternative treatment?** | Oral contraceptives 4 times a day for 1 week, then begin normal regimen for at least 3 months |

## BREAST

CASE 7

*A 38-year-old female presents with a palpable breast lump that she detected while showering. She denies any nipple discharge, bone pain, or abnormality in the breast's appearance.*

| | |
|---|---|
| **What are you most concerned about?** | Breast cancer |
| **How does it commonly present?** | Palpable painless mass or an abnormal mammogram without a palpable mass |
| **What risk factors should be questioned?** | Family history (first-degree relatives), early menarche, late menopause, nullparity and first pregnancy after age 30, and previous breast cancer or biopsies with atypical changes |
| **What physical exam findings suggest breast cancer?** | Color change, dimpling, nipple retraction, axillary mass, and bone pain (rare) |
| **What test should be ordered first?** | Mammogram |
| **What findings on mammogram suggest breast cancer?** | Clustered microcalcifications and stellate densities |
| **How is the diagnosis confirmed?** | Biopsy (excisional, incisional, or fine needle) |
| **What's the treatment for Stage I or II?** | Either modified radical mastectomy or lumpectomy followed by radiation; axillary lymph node sampling |
| **Locally advanced (stage III)?** | Combination chemotherapy and radiation therapy prior to mastectomy |
| **Metastatic (stage IV) disease?** | Combinations of chemotherapy, hormone therapy, and radiation therapy |

## COMPLICATED PREGNANCY

### CASE 8

*A 25-year-old female in third trimester of pregnancy develops severe abdominal pain and vaginal bleeding after being struck in the abdomen by her abusive husband.*

| | |
|---|---|
| **What complication should you be concerned about?** | Abruptio placenta |
| **What is it?** | Separation of a normally implanted placenta from the uterine wall |
| **How does it classically present?** | Third trimester bleeding with severe abdominal pain |
| **What principal risk factor does she have?** | Trauma |
| **What other risk factors should be investigated?** | Hypertension, cigarettes, cocaine, and previous abruption |
| **What physical exam findings support the diagnosis?** | Firm tender uterus with or without signs of fetal distress |
| **What labs should be ordered?** | Type and screen, CBC, coagulation studies, fibrinogen level, and cocaine drug screen |
| **What imaging test should be ordered?** | Abdominal ultrasound |
| **How is the diagnosis made?** | Clinical history and presentation |
| **How is the diagnosis confirmed?** | Examination of placenta after delivery |
| **What is the treatment if mother and fetus are stable?** | Bed rest with a fetal monitor |
| **What is the treatment for uncontrollable hemorrhaging or maternal or fetal compromise?** | Immediate cesarean section |

## CASE 9

*A 24-year-old female with history of PID presents with acute onset of right lower quadrant abdominal pain and vaginal spotting. Prior to the abrupt onset of pain, she had some crampy abdominal pain, nausea, and rare spotting. Her menses is now 3 weeks late.*

**What do you suspect?**

Ectopic pregnancy (fertilized ovum implants outside the uterus) with possible rupture

**Why?**

Amenorrhea, nausea, spotting, and crampy lower abdominal pain are characteristic of an ectopic pregnancy.

**What symptoms are worrisome for rupture?**

Rapid onset of severe sharp abdominal or pelvic pain, guarding, rigidity, rebound tenderness, and vaginal bleeding; hypotension and shock may be present.

**What risk factor does she have?**

PID

**What other risk factors should be questioned?**

Intrauterine device (IUD), tubal surgery, and prior ectopic pregnancy

**What physical exam findings support the diagnosis?**

Tender abdomen and adnexae; adnexal mass may be appreciated

**What lab tests should be ordered?**

CBC, blood type, antibody screen and crossmatch, quantitative $\beta$-hCG level

**What lab result supports the diagnosis?**

A $\beta$-hCG level that fails to double in 48 hours and lack of gestational sac in utero

**If pregnancy test is positive, what radiographic study should be ordered next?**

Transvaginal or transabdominal ultrasound (may reveal empty uterine cavity and an adnexal mass)

**How is the diagnosis confirmed?**

Laparoscopy

**What medical treatment should all Rh-negative women receive?**

Rhogam

**What are the treatment options for unruptured ectopic pregnancies if detected early?**

Methotrexate, laparoscopic tubal surgery or salpingectomy

| | |
|---|---|
| **What is the treatment for a ruptured ectopic pregnancy?** | Laparoscopic salpingectomy or salpingostomy after patient is stabilized |

## CASE 10

*A 26-year-old female with 3 prior abortions now in her third trimester of an uncomplicated pregnancy presents with intermittent painless bright red vaginal bleeding. Over the last 4 days it has occurred twice and only soaked 3 pads. She denies any abdominal pain, trauma, or drug use. She is still able to feel the baby kick as before.*

| | |
|---|---|
| **What should you be concerned about?** | Placenta previa |
| **Why?** | Sudden onset of painless bright red third-trimester vaginal bleeding; often resolves spontaneously and reoccurs days later |
| **Where does the placenta lie in placenta previa?** | Over or near the cervical os |
| **What is her known risk factor?** | Prior abortions |
| **What are the other risk factors?** | Multiparity, advanced maternal age, and previous cesarean section |
| **Should a vaginal exam be conducted during the physical exam?** | No, it may cause increased bleeding |
| **What basic labs should be ordered?** | CBC, blood type, blood screen, and coagulation studies |
| **How is it diagnosed?** | Transabdominal or transvaginal ultrasound |
| **What is the treatment for placenta previa with minor bleeding?** | Bed rest, tocolytics if necessary, and delivery by cesarean section |
| **What is the treatment for placenta previa with severe bleeding?** | Stabilize mother and immediate cesarean section |

## CASE 11

*A 26-year-old G3P3 female with history of hypertension presents to the ER with progressive onset of headache, blurred vision, nausea, and vomiting. Her current blood pressure is 170/90.*

| | |
|---|---|
| **What diagnosis do you suspect?** | Preeclampsia (pregnancy-induced hypertension) |
| **What's its classic presentation?** | Headache, blurred vision, scotomata, edema, nausea, and vomiting |
| **What are the risk factors?** | Multiple gestation and preexisting hypertension |
| **What other risk factors are there?** | Molar pregnancy and age |
| **What findings may be apparent on physical exam?** | Hypertension, generalized nondependent edema, and oliguria |
| **What will the urinalysis reveal?** | Proteinuria |
| **How is hypertension defined in pregnancy?** | A blood pressure >140/90 or a 30 mm Hg increase in systolic or 15 mm Hg increase in diastolic during pregnancy |
| **How is mild preeclampsia diagnosed?** | Hypertension with nondependent edema or 2+ proteinuria |
| **How is severe preeclampsia diagnosed?** | Blood pressure of 160/110, oliguria, 3+ proteinuria, or evidence of end organ damage |
| **How is eclampsia diagnosed?** | Seizure activity in a preeclamptic patient |
| **What is the treatment goal?** | Avoid complications of end organ damage and eclampsia |
| **How is mild preeclampsia treated?** | Bed rest with decreased water intake; induce delivery if fetus is full term and use IV magnesium for seizure prophylaxis |

| How are severe preeclampsia and eclampsia treated? | Deliver baby after mother has been stabilized, may use antihypertensive medications like hydralazine, use magnesium for seizure prophylaxis, and add IV diazepam if seizures develop |

## MISCELLANEOUS CONDITIONS

### CASE 12

*A 22-year-old female in her 17th week of pregnancy presents to your office concerned about vaginal spotting and uterine cramping.*

| What are you concerned about? | Spontaneous abortion (SAB) (spontaneous loss of a pregnancy before 20 weeks gestation) |
| What is the main cause in first-trimester SAB? | Fetal chromosomal abnormalities |
| What are some common causes of second trimester SAB? | Maternal infections, cervical incompetence, uterine anomalies, endocrine abnormalities, systemic disease, and environmental factors (e.g., smoking, alcohol, and cocaine) |
| What should be included in the workup to assess maternal and fetal well being? | Maternal vital signs and fetal heart rate |
| What lab tests should be ordered? | β-hCG, CBC, type and screen, and PTT |
| What radiographic study is helpful to determine viable pregnancies? | Transvaginal or transabdominal ultrasound |
| Describe the exam findings in the different types of SABs:<br>  **Threatened abortion** | Cervical os is closed |
|   **Inevitable abortion** | Cervix is dilated or membranes have ruptured |

| | |
|---|---|
| **Incomplete abortion** | Dilated cervix with some of the products of conception passing through the cervix |
| **Complete abortion** | All products of conception have passed through the cervix |
| **Missed abortion** | Retention of failed intrauterine pregnancy for at least 4 weeks |
| **How is an abortion diagnosed?** | History, presentation, speculum exam findings, and ultrasound if needed |

**What is the treatment for the different types of abortions?**

| | |
|---|---|
| **Threatened** | Maternal bed rest and pelvic rest for stable mothers with a viable fetus |
| **Inevitable** | Either wait for the abortion to complete or perform a dilation and curettage (D&C) |
| **Incomplete** | D&C |
| **Missed** | D&C (preferred) or await spontaneous abortion (risk of hemorrhage) |

# 11 Pediatrics

## GASTROENTEROLOGY

CASE 1

*A previously healthy 20-day-old infant is brought to your office by his exhausted parents complaining that their child has been crying most days for the last week with his legs drawn up toward his belly.*

| | |
|---|---|
| **What differential diagnosis are you considering?** | Bone fracture, physical abuse, incarcerated hernia, milk or formula intolerance, corneal abrasion, and colic |
| **You've completed a thorough physical exam and other than the child crying excessively and the abdomen being slightly distended, he appears to be healthy. What is your most likely diagnosis?** | Colic |
| **Why?** | Healthy child with normal physical exam crying excessively for more than 3 hours per day for 3 days a week during 1st 3 months of life is diagnostic of colic. |
| **Why does this not fit formula or milk intolerance?** | Lack of diarrhea or vomiting |
| **What causes colic?** | Unknown |
| **What treatment should you begin?** | Carry and cuddle baby when crying, supportive counseling (this is nothing you have done to the baby), and parental reassurance (it's going to get better) |
| **Are there any medications to prescribe?** | No |
| **When do most cases of colic resolve?** | By 3 months |

## CASE 2

*A 2-week-old infant presents with progressively worse projectile nonbilious vomiting after meals for the last 3 days.*

| | |
|---|---|
| **What's your differential diagnosis?** | Gastroenteritis, pyloric stenosis, urinary tract infection (UTI), formula intolerance, drug withdrawal, gastric or duodenal web |
| **On physical exam you find a firm, 1–2 cm "olive" 2 or 3 cm above the umbilicus with a visible peristaltic wave over the epigastrium. What just came to the top of your DDx?** | Pyloric stenosis |
| **What does the olive represent?** | Hypertrophied pylorus |
| **Before ordering your diagnostic test, you need to order what lab test?** | Chem 8 to check for hypochloremic hypokalemic metabolic alkalosis secondary to excess gastric fluid loss |
| **Your chemistries come back within normal limits. What diagnostic test do you want to order?** | Abdominal ultrasound (90–100% sensitive, best diagnostic test) |
| **The ultrasound comes back with the result of poor study owing to patient movement. What is the next test you order?** | Upper GI study |
| **Report comes back stating findings are consistent with pyloric stenosis. What causes it?** | Hypertrophy of the circular muscle of the pylorus causing gastric outlet obstruction |
| **At what age does it usually present?** | 1–10 weeks |

| | |
|---|---|
| **What is the incidence?** | 3 per 100 live births |
| **Is there a gender bias?** | Yes. Males are affected four times as often as females. |
| **Is there a racial bias?** | Yes. Whites are the most frequently affected, followed by African Americans. Orientals and Indians are rarely affected. |
| **Does birth order play a role?** | Yes. First-born children are the most frequently affected. |
| **What is the treatment of choice?** | Pylorotomy |
| **Is this curative?** | Yes |

CASE 3

*A 6-month-old boy presents with recurrent and severe paroxysmal colicky abdominal pain, emesis, loud cries, and bloody mucus stools. The emesis was initially clear, but has become bile stained prior to presentation.*

| | |
|---|---|
| **What is your differential diagnosis?** | Adhesions causing small bowel obstruction (SBO), intussusception, gastroenteritis, appendicitis |
| **You examine the child and find an oblong sausage-shaped palpable mass in the right upper quadrant (RUQ) or mid-epigastric area and currant jelly-appearing stool. What do you think the diagnosis is now?** | Intussusception |
| **Why?** | Triad of colicky abdominal pain, emesis, currant jelly stools, and palpable RUQ mass in age-appropriate child (usually 3 months to 6 years, 66% before 1st year) and this is the most common cause of intestinal obstruction in this age group |

| | |
|---|---|
| **What basic labs and tests should you order?** | Chem 8, CBC, UA, stool guaiac |
| **What imaging test will suggest the diagnosis?** | Plain x-ray showing a soft tissue mass that displaces the gas-filled bowel with or without evidence of bowel obstruction |
| **Does a normal x-ray rule out intussusception?** | No |
| **What test will you order to make the diagnosis?** | An air or barium enema done under fluoroscopic guidance |
| **What do you expect it to show?** | Filling defect at the distal end of the intussusception giving a "coiled spring" appearance |
| **What causes it?** | A telescoping of part of the intestine into a segment distal to itself |
| **What is the primary site of intussusception?** | 95% of cases are ileocolic, beginning just proximal to the cecum. |
| **What gives the coiled spring appearance on barium enema?** | It occurs when contrast fills the space between the intussusceptum and the intussuscipiens. |
| **What causes this?** | Usually, no cause is found. There is an association with adenoviruses and gastroenteritis. Other causes include Meckel diverticulum, intestinal polyps, and Henoch-Schönlein purpura. |
| **How does a lead point such as a Meckel diverticulum cause intususception?** | It has been suggested that the lead point, such as a Meckel diverticulum or swollen Peyer patches from infection, stimulates the ileum to contract in an attempt to extrude the mass and thus causes an intussusception. |
| **What causes the abdominal pain?** | Peristalsis pulling on the intussusceptum. As peristalsis is an on-and-off phenomenon, so the pain initially comes and goes, and children are fine in between spells. |

When they have the pain, younger children will usually pull up their knees and strain.

**Why does bleeding occur?**

The intestine pulls the mesentery along with itself, constricting it. This leads to venous pooling and edema of the mucosa, followed by bleeding.

**How is this treated?**

Barium enema (the diagnostic test); the pressure of the enema is usually sufficient to reduce the intussusception.

**What if this fails?**

Surgery

## CASE 4

A concerned mother calls you because her 3-year-old child has been acting strangely since visiting his grandmother this morning who has multiple medical conditions requiring numerous medications. The grandma complained to the mother earlier that the boy had spilled all her medications in her pill box on the floor. For the last 15 minutes, the child has begun to salivate, has watery eyes, urinated on himself, and has thrown up in the back seat of the car.

**What are you most concerned about?**

Poisoning

**Who's at greatest risk of poisoning?**

Children <5 years old

**When should a diagnosis of poisoning be considered?**

In a patient with a known or suspected exposure to a toxin, or in an individual with the sudden onset of mental status changes, respiratory aberrations, abnormal behavior, shock, autonomic dysfunction, vomiting and/or diarrhea, dysrhythmia, or metabolic derangements not otherwise explained

**What does the mother need to do first?**

Take the child to the ER.

**What four types of poisoning syndromes should you be considering in this child?**

Cholinergic, anticholinergic, sympathomimetic, sympatholytic

**How does cholinergic syndrome present, and what drugs cause this?**

This comes from stimulation of muscarinic and nicotinic receptors. The mnemonic **SLUDGE** is helpful here: **S**alivation, **L**acrimation, **U**rination, **D**efecation, **G**I cramps, and **E**mesis. Pupils are constricted. Drugs that cause this include organophosphates, physostigmine, and nicotine.

**How does anticholinergic syndrome present, and what drugs cause this?**

"Mad as a hatter, hot as a hare, dry as a bone, red as a beet." Tachycardia and hypertension are also seen, and pupils are dilated. Drugs to consider are atropine, scopolamine, cyclic antidepressants, jimsonweed, antihistamines, and *Amanita muscaria* poisoning.

**How does sympathomimetic syndrome present, and what drugs cause this?**

Heart rate and blood pressure are increased, and the temperature is elevated. The patient is diaphoretic, pupils are dilated, the mouth is dry, and he is frequently agitated. Drugs include amphetamines, cocaine, phencyclidine, pseudoephedrine, caffeine, methylphenidate, and theophylline.

**How does sympatholytic syndrome present, and what drugs cause this?**

As expected, this is the opposite of sympathomimetic. Affected patients have bradycardia, hypotension, and hypothermia. The skin is dry, pupils constricted, and bowel sounds may be absent. There may be signs of central nervous system depression. Think of opioids, alcohol, heroin, barbiturates, benzodiazapines, and clonidine.

**Which type does this child most likely have?**

Cholinergic

**What labs should you order?**

CMP, CBC, urine, and serum drug screen

How do urine and ser[um]
toxicology screens differ?

What therapy should this
child receive?

Ipe[cac]
activate[d]

When should emesis not be
induced?

Coma, conv[ulsions]
antidepressants,
(The 5 C's.)

What additional measure
may be used?

Gastric lavage

What are the limitations of
gastric lavage?

The ingestion must be recent (w[ithin]
2 hours) and the patient must be ab[le to]
protect his airway (i.e., no depression [of]
sensorium or potential of seizure).

When should activated
charcoal not be used?

If there is a possibility of endoscopy,
drugs for which there is an oral antidote,
hydrocarbons, and those that do not adsorb
to it, including heavy metals, lithium, iron,
acids, alkalis, alcohols, and cyanide

What additional measures
should be taken at grandma's
house?

Keep medications and other toxic
substances out of reach by using child-
proof cabinets, drawers, and medicine
bottles.

## HEAD AND NECK INFECTIONS

### CASE 5

*A 24-month-old toddler is brought to the walk-in clinic with persistent crying
and inability to be calmed for last 18 hours. The mother says that since yesterday the child has been pulling on his right ear and crying. She has taken
his temperature and it was 37.7°C. Tylenol has not worked and she wants to
know what can be done next. She later informs you that last week he had
some clear nasal discharge, but it has significantly decreased over the last
few days.*

media)

ng with
a classic
dia

of fullness
the

fever,

y infection

oviruses,
ases

Urine screens are designed primarily
for drugs of abuse, while serum tests
are for over-the-counter products and
alcohol.

ac syrup to induce vomiting, and
d charcoal to help absorb toxin

sions, caustics, cyclic
and hydrocarbons

thin 1 to
le to
of

**What are the 3 most common bacterial causes of AOM?**

*Streptococcus pneumonia, Hemophilus influenzae, Moraxella catarrhalis*

**What clinical findings on otoscopy of AOM do you expect to find?**

Injection, erythema, loss of luster of tympanic membrane, loss of translucency of some or all or membrane, bulging of membrane or loss of landmarks

**Is erythema diagnostic of AOM?**

No, erythema may be caused by inflammation of mucosa throughout the upper respiratory tract.

**How is the diagnosis made?**

Pneumatic otoscopy, with or without tympanometry

**What is the treatment strategy for AOM?**

Oral antibiotics for 10 days

**What are first-line treatment options?**

Amoxicillin, or trimethoprim-sulfamethoxazole (TMP-SMZ) for penicillin-allergic persons

| | |
|---|---|
| **What are the typical doses of amoxicillin and TMP-SMZ used?** | Amoxicillin 250–500 mg by mouth 3 times a day, or TMP-SMZ 1 tablet by mouth twice a day |
| **What medication can be used to treat pain and fever?** | Children's Tylenol |

## CASE 6

*A 12-year-old boy presents to the clinic with a 2-week history of frontal headache accompanied by nasal drainage. The child said at first the drainage was clear and accompanied by a cough, but has now turned a dark yellow color with brown streaks. He has been taking antihistamines for his allergies and over-the-counter Tylenol, but it has not helped. His mother wants to know if it's time for an antibiotic.*

| | |
|---|---|
| **What is this child's presentation consistent with?** | Acute sinusitis |
| **What is acute sinusitis?** | Inflammation of the mucosal lining of the paranasal sinuses, lasting up to 3 weeks. |
| **Where does the infection most likely reside in this child?** | Frontal sinus |
| **Why?** | He complains of a frontal headache. |
| **What other sinuses can be involved in acute sinusitis?** | Maxillary, ethmoid, sphenoid |
| **What type of acute sinusitis did this child have initially?** | Acute viral sinusitis |
| **How does viral sinusitis most commonly present?** | Nasal drainage and cough |
| **What other signs and symptoms commonly occur with it?** | Fever and sore throat |

**What are the common agents in viral sinusitis?**

Rhinovirus, coronavirus, influenza, parainfluenza, adenovirus, enterovirus, and respiratory syncytial virus

**What is the most likely explanation for the recent change in nasal discharge?**

Superimposed acute bacterial rhinosinusitis (ABRS)

**Define it.**

Sinusitis with bacterial superinfection

**What is the major risk factor for developing ABRS?**

Viral sinusitis for more than 7–10 days (which he had)

**What are the two most common bacterial agents in ABRS?**

*Streptococcus pneumoniae* and nontypable *Hemophilus influenzae*

**What other pathogens may cause ABRS?**

*Moraxella catarrhalis,* other streptococcal species, anaerobic bacteria, and *Staphylococcus aureus*

**How does ABRS most commonly present?**

Purulent nasal drainage and sinus pressure or tenderness

**What other signs and symptoms may occur?**

Fever is present in about one-half of cases. Sinus pain may be worse when bending or supine.

**What is the gold standard for the diagnosis of ABRS?**

Sinus puncture with culture of the aspirated fluid

**How is a clinical diagnosis of ABRS made?**

Vancomycin resistant streptococci (VRS) present >10 days (or worsens after 5–7 days) and is accompanied by some of the following symptoms: nasal drainage, nasal congestion, facial pain/pressure (particularly with unilateral predominance), postnasal drainage, fever, cough, fatigue, hyposmia/anosmia, maxillary dental pain, ear pressure/fullness.

**What is the treatment strategy for ABRS?**

Oral antibiotics for at least 10 days

**What are first-line treatment options for mild to moderate disease in a β-lactam nonallergic adult with no recent antibiotic exposure?**

"High-dose" amoxicillin, amoxicillin/ clavulanic acid, cefpodoxime, or cefuroxime axetil

**What first-line antibiotic options are recommended for a β-lactam allergic patient with mild to moderate disease?**

TMP-SMZ, doxycycline, or a macrolide (e.g., clarithromycin, azithromycin)

## CASE 7

*A 15-year-old boy complains of rapid onset of severe sore throat, fever of 38°C, and mild headache. The physical exam provided by the school nurse notes anterior cervical adenopathy and red posterior pharynx with white exudates.*

**What's the most likely diagnosis?**

Exudative pharyngitis

**Define it.**

Inflammation of the pharynx, presenting with sore throat and tonsillopharyngeal exudate

**What's the most common cause of pharyngitis?**

Viruses

**Which viruses can cause exudative pharyngitis?**

Epstein-Barr virus (infectious mononucleosis), herpes simplex virus, and adenovirus

**What additional clinical findings would suggest Epstein-Barr virus infection?**

Fatigue, malaise, and prominent cervical adenopathy (particularly posterior cervical). Exudate is seen in one-half of cases and palatal petechiae are seen in 25%. Splenomegaly may also occur.

**What office-based laboratory test can help establish the diagnosis of infectious mononucleosis as a result of Epstein-Barr virus?**

The "spot" test for heterophile antibodies (the monospot test)

| | |
|---|---|
| **Name three bacterial causes of pharyngitis.** | *Streptococcus pyogenes, Neisseria gonorrhoeae, Corynebacterium diphtheriae* |
| **Why should group A β-hemolytic streptococcus (GABHS) be treated?** | Prevention of suppurative complications and prevention of rheumatic fever |
| **What are the suppurative complications of GABHS pharyngitis?** | Peritonsillar or retropharyngeal abscess, otitis media, mastoiditis, sinusitis, and suppurative cervical lymphadenitis |
| **What clinical findings increase the likelihood that pharyngitis is due to GABHS?** | Tonsillar exudates; swollen, tender, anterior cervical lymph nodes; history of fever; absence of cough |
| **What office-based laboratory testing is available for the diagnosis of GABHS?** | Rapid antigen detection tests and throat culture |
| **Does a negative rapid antigen detection test rule out GABHS?** | No. Rapid antigen detection tests have a sensitivity of approximately 85%; therefore, the diagnosis cannot be ruled out with certainty on the basis of a negative test. |
| **What is the gold standard diagnostic test in GABHS?** | Throat culture |
| **When should one order the throat culture?** | Negative rapid antigen detection test with a high index of clinical suspicion for GABHS |
| **If the rapid antigen test is positive for GABHS, is throat culture required?** | No |
| **What is the treatment of choice for pharyngitis as a result of GABHS?** | Oral penicillin for 10 days |
| **What treatment is recommended for GABHS in patients with penicillin allergy?** | Erythromycin |

## INFECTIOUS DISEASES

### CASE 8

*A 4-year-old girl presents from day care with her mother to your clinic in December with a 3-day history of nonbloody diarrhea preceded by multiple episodes of vomiting.*

**What broad differential diagnosis are you considering?**

| | |
|---|---|
| **Viral** | Enterovirus, rotavirus, adenovirus, and Norwalk virus |
| **Bacterial** | *Salmonella, Shigella, Yersinia, Campylobacter* and enteroinvasive *Escherichia coli, Staphylococcus,* and *Clostridium difficile* |

**Is viral or bacterial cause more likely here?**

Viral for 2 reasons: first, viral is the most common cause of diarrhea in children (70–80%). Second, vomiting preceded the diarrhea and no blood or mucous is described with the diarrhea, which is more consistent with a viral cause.

**Which bacterial organism should you keep in your differential diagnosis?**

*Staphlococcus,* because it also produces both vomiting and diarrhea

**What clue in the presentation helps narrow down your differential diagnosis for the causative virus?**

Season of the year

**Name the most common virus in**

| | |
|---|---|
| **Winter (in this case) and spring** | Rotavirus |
| **Summer** | Enterovirus |

**Name other causative viruses not associated with a particular season.**

Adenovirus and Norwalk virus

**What then is the most likely cause of this patient's diarrhea?**

Rotavirus

**Pertinent positive physical exam findings include pulse of 130, respiratory rate of 24, dry mucus membranes, 2-pound weight loss from last clinic visit, and stool heme. What do these findings suggest?**

Dehydration (yes) and viral etiology (no blood in stool)

**What basic lab tests should be considered to strengthen your diagnosis?**

CBC with differential (WBC high in invasive infectious process), Chem 8 (check of evidence of dehydration and acid–base imbalance from diarrhea with or without vomiting), blood cultures (if suspect bacteremia)

**What presenting sign and symptom would make you suspect bacteremia?**

Fever, chills

**What are the stool diagnostic tests of choice?**

Stool culture and Gram stain, fecal PMN count, and fecal occult blood test

**What are the associated lab findings for bacterial organisms?**

Positive fecal occult blood with numerous PMNs

**What additional tests can be ordered to confirm a viral etiology?**

Rotazyme assay (if rotavirus suspected, winter), ELISA test for suspected virus

**What is the treatment strategy for both viral and bacterial gastroenteritis?**

Supportive with oral rehydration as needed

| When is antibiotic use indicated? | *Shigella* infections and other bacterial gastroenteritis that is failing conservative treatment |
|---|---|
| What antibiotic is recommended to treat *Shigella* and many other bacterial organisms causing gastroenteritis? | Bactrim |
| Are antidiarrheal medications (e.g., Lomotil, Imodium) recommended? | No |

## CASE 9

*A concerned mother brings her 2-year-old child 2 weeks after a family reunion with 12 other cousins with a new rash preceded by a low-grade fever, lack of appetite, and decreased playful activity. She states the rash began on the face and trunk, then spread to the extremities. The rash began as small, round, flat or raised red areas then progressed to small pruritic vesicles with clear fluid.*

| What differential diagnosis should you consider? | Chicken pox (Varicella-Zoster virus), Coxsackie virus, disseminated herpes simplex virus, echovirus, and atypical measles |
|---|---|
| What question should you ask her about the family reunion? | Did any of the children have a similar rash? |
| She informs you that her cousin's son had small, clear vesicles on his face, hands, and arms. What diagnosis do you suspect? | Chicken pox caused by the Varicella-Zoster virus |
| Why? | Sick contact 10–20 days ago, prodrome and constitutional symptoms, rash began on face and trunk and spread to extremities, started maculopapular to vesicular |

| | |
|---|---|
| **What test can you order to confirm your clinical suspicion?** | Tzanck smear *Fluid from Vesicle stained or slide. Multinucleated Giant Cells* |
| **What treatment can you offer?** | Diphenhydramine (pruritis) and acetaminophen (fever) |

## CASE 10

*A 4-year-old newly adopted child from a developing country recently immigrant presents with malaise, fever of 102°F, conjunctivitis, cough and runny nose, and a rash. The rash began on the head and progressed caudally to the trunk and extremities. On exam it appears confluent, erythematous, and maculopapular.*

| | |
|---|---|
| **What is your differential diagnosis?** | Kawasaki syndrome, infectious mononucleosis, scarlet fever, toxoplasmosis, drug eruption, and mycoplasma pneumonia |
| **On exam you identify small blue-white punctate spots with whitish centers on the buccal mucosa. What are these called?** | Koplik spots |
| **What is your diagnosis now?** | Measles (rubeola) with the 3 C's—cough, coryza, and conjunctivitis |
| **Why?** | Because these buccal spots are pathognomonic for measles |
| **How could the diagnosis be confirmed?** | ELISA test (rarely done) |
| **What causes measles?** | Paramyxovirus |
| **How is it transmitted?** | Respiratory secretions |
| **What most likely put this child at risk of contracting the illness?** | Inadequate immunizations in the developing country |
| **What is the treatment?** | Supportive (rest, oral rehydration, and acetaminophen for fever) |

CASE 11

*In a rural town within a developing country you see a 6-year old-boy with fever, malaise, headache, abdominal pain, and swollen neck. On exam you find bilaterally swollen parotid glands.*

| | |
|---|---|
| **What's your differential diagnosis?** | Mostly viral agents (paramyxovirus, influenza A, Coxsackie virus, parainfluenza, HIV), diabetes, uremia, and drugs |
| **What's the most likely cause in this child?** | Paramyxovirus (mumps) |
| **How do you make the diagnosis?** | By history and physical exam |
| **Which elevated serum chemistry tests would support your diagnosis?** | Elevated amylase and lipase |
| **How can the diagnosis be confirmed?** | ELISA test for paramyxovirus (rarely done) |
| **Why is this disease uncommon in the United States?** | Proper immunization of children protects against contracting the illness. |
| **How do unimmunized children spread the virus?** | Nasopharyngeal secretions |
| **What are children with mumps at risk for?** | Pancreatitis, meningitis, encephalitis, hearing loss, and orchitis (in pubescent males) |
| **What is the treatment?** | Supportive (oral rehydration and acetaminophen as needed) |
| **How long will the illness last on average?** | 1 week |

CASE 12

*A recently illegally immigrated mother brings her 18-month-old child in with a rash. 1–5 days prior to the rash the child had low-grade fever, cough, conjunctivitis, coryza, malaise, headache, and lymphadenopathy for 1–5 days. The rash began on the head and progressed to the trunk and extremities. On exam it appears erythematous and maculopapular.*

| | |
|---|---|
| **What is your differential diagnosis?** | Measles (both rubella, rubeola), scarlet fever, infectious mononucleosis, toxoplasmosis, erythema infectiosum, drug rash |
| **What is the significance of immigration?** | Suspect incomplete immunization record |
| **What 2 illnesses top your differential diagnosis?** | Measles (both rubella, rubeola) |
| **To help distinguish between the two, you go back to examine the patient's rash and one finding solidifies your diagnosis. What did you notice?** | The rash does not coalesce, which is different from coalescing rash seen in rubella (measles). |
| **What's your diagnosis now?** | Rubella (German measles) |
| **You've made a tentative diagnosis based on history and presentation. How can you confirm it?** | Increase in serum antibodies to rubella virus |
| **How is it treated?** | Supportive (most spontaneously resolve); NSAIDs (acetaminophen) for fever |
| **Is this child contagious?** | Yes, for 1 week before and after onset of rash |
| **So what additional measures should you take?** | Do not expose patient to unimmunized individuals (especially pregnant women) 1 week before or after onset of rash. |
| **Which viral agent causes it?** | Togavirus |
| **How was it transmitted?** | Airborne nasopharyngeal droplets or transplacental passage to fetus |

| | |
|---|---|
| **Who is at greatest risk of contracting the illness?** | Fetuses of unimmunized pregnant women in the first and second trimesters |
| **What increases the risk in adolescents and adults?** | Inadequate MMR vaccination as a child |
| **If this child had been a neonate of an unimmunized mother, how would he have presented?** | Congenital anomalies (over 50%) with risk of hydrops fetalis |
| **If an unimmunized pregnant women is exposed to togovirus, should she be immunized?** | No, rubella immunization is contraindicated during pregnancy. |

## CASE 13

*A mother brings her 7-year-old boy in for once-weekly bedwetting and infrequent wet daytime pants for the last 4 months.*

| | |
|---|---|
| **What's your differential diagnosis?** | Primary enuresis; secondary enuresis to ADH deficiency (rare), diabetes mellitus (DM), urinary tract infection (UTI), obstruction, and developmental delay |
| **If this child were 4 years old, would you be concerned?** | No, because some boys take up to 6 years old to control their bladders (5 years old for girls). |
| **If this child were having incontinence only once every 5 weeks, would it be considered abnormal?** | No, it is a problem when it occurs more than once a month. |
| **What lab tests should you order?** | UA (detects UTI and DM) and culture |
| **Labs and culture come back normal (no UTI or DM). What is your diagnosis?** | Primary enuresis |

| | |
|---|---|
| **What's the treatment?** | Use of a nighttime audio alarm that sounds when child urinates (assists bladder control conditioning) |
| **The mother comes back for 2 successive follow-ups and the problem persists. What's your next step?** | Consider medical therapy with imipramine (tricyclic antidepressant) or intranasal desmopressin acetate (an endogenous vasopressin analog). |
| **What risks are associated with imipramine therapy?** | Arrhythmias, conduction blocks, accidental overdose, and death |
| **What study should be ordered prior to starting a child on imipramine?** | EKG |

## CASE 14

*A previously healthy 1-year-old child comes to the emergency room in November with a 3-day history of mild cold symptoms including runny nose, slight cough, and feeling hot. Over the last 24 hours, the child's cough has worsened and breathing is slightly more labored, but he is still breast-feeding well. On exam you find low-grade fever, mild tachypnea, and soft expiratory wheezing.*

| | |
|---|---|
| **What differential diagnosis should you be considering?** | Viral bronchiolitis, asthma, vascular ring, foreign body, congenital heart disease, pneumonia, reflux, aspiration, croup, and cystic fibrosis |
| **What tests should you consider ordering?** | CBC, serum electrolytes, urinalysis, pulse oximetry measurement, and CXR |
| **All tests are normal except for mild leukocytosis and peribronchial thickening on CXR. What is your most likely diagnosis?** | Respiratory syncytial virus (RSV) bronchiolitis |
| **What can you order to confirm your diagnosis?** | Immunofluorescent or enzyme immunoassay detection of RSV antigen of suctioned nasal secretions |

| | |
|---|---|
| **What severity of RSV bronchiolitis does this child have?** | Mild |
| **What is the management of mild RSV bronchiolitis?** | Home with supportive treatment, oral hydration, and nasal suctioning |
| **48 hours later the mother brings the child back with significant wheezing, tachypnea, fever, nasal flaring, retractions, cyanosis, decreased air entry, and prolonged expiratory phase with wheezing. Your prior diagnosis of RSV bronchiolitis is confirmed by lab review and the prior lab panel and CXR is ordered. What should you do first?** | $O_2$ supplementation, pulse ox monitoring (observation for apnea and respiratory failure), ABG (due to cyanosis), inhaled bronchodilators such as albuterol or racemic epinephrine can be tried cautiously, IV hydration, Tylenol |
| **Would corticosteroids or antibiotics be helpful?** | No |
| **What should you do once you've stabilized the patient?** | Order CBC, chem 8, ua, blood culture, and CXR |
| **Labs confirm infection (leukocytosis), dehydration (elevated BUN/cr), and mild hypoxia, and radiographic imaging confirms worsened parenchymal disease. Should this patient be discharged with supportive care?** | No, hospital admission is warranted. |
| **What are some hospital admission criteria for patients with RSV bronchiolitis?** | Children with dehydration, poor oral intake, significant respiratory distress, hypoxia, and apnea |
| **What complication did this patient have?** | Respiratory failure and atrial tachycardia |
| **What additional complications are there?** | Pneumonia and apnea |

**What additional investigations should be considered during hospitalization?**

Risk factors for severe RSV bronchiolitis

**What are they?**

Premature birth, chronic lung disease (CLD), bronchopulmonary dysplasia, cystic fibrosis, congenital heart disease, and immunodeficiency

**What is the mechanism of disease for viral bronchiolitis?**

Viral inflammation of the small airways resulting in necrosis of the respiratory epithelium, obstruction of the airway lumen, and leukocyte peribronchial infiltration causing edema of the bronchiolar wall

**What are the causes of viral bronchiolitis?**

RSV is the most common cause. Other less common viruses include influenza, parainfluenza, and adenovirus.

**How do RSV infections occur in the Northern Hemisphere?**

In epidemics between October and April of each year.

**What age groups are most susceptible to RSV bronchiolitis?**

Children younger than 2 years of age

**What control measures should be taken to minimize spread of RSV infection to susceptible children in the hospital?**

Segregation of infected infants and staff is required. Infected children should be placed in contact isolation and the use of gowns, gloves, and strict hand washing should be observed.

**How could RSV bronchiolitis be prevented?**

RSV immune globulin intravenous (RSV-IGIV) and Palivizumab are 2 drugs that were produced by the same manufacturer and have been approved for the prevention of RSV infection. Either monthly intravenous RSV-IGIV or monthly intramuscular Palivizumab is given during the RSV season for a total of 5 treatments.

**Who should be given RSV-IGIV or Palivizumab?**

Children younger than 2 years of age with CLD who required treatment for CLD within 6 months before the start of their first RSV season. Infants born before 32 weeks of gestation with or without CLD may benefit from prophylaxis based on the gestational age at birth, chronological age at the start of the first RSV season, and their community RSV bronchiolitis rehospitalization data.

## CASE 15

**When a child comes to your office with a chief complaint of sore throat, what is your broad differential diagnosis?**

Pharyngitis

    **Viral?**

Adenovirus (most common), Coxsackie, Epstein-Barr virus (EBV), influenza, rhinovirus, parainfluenza, RSV, measles, rubella, HIV, and herpes simplex

    **Bacterial?**

Group A β-hemolytic *Streptococcus* (GABHS) (*Streptococcus pyogenes*) (most common agent), *Mycoplasma pneumoniae*, group G and C streptococci, *Arcanobacterium hemolyticum*, *Corynebacterium diphtheriae*, *C. hemolyticum*, *Neisseria gonorrhea*, *N. meningitidis*, *Francisella tularensis*, *Treponema pallidum*, oropharyngeal anaerobes, and *Chlamydia pneumoniae*

**For each risk factor below (presentation clue to pay attention to), name the associated agent known to cause pharyngitis.**

    **Overcrowding**

*Streptococcus* species

    **Sexual activity**

*N. gonorrhea, T. pallidum*, EBV

| | |
|---|---|
| **Swimming in an inadequately chlorinated pool** | Adenovirus |
| **Eating undercooked meat** | Tularemia |
| **Incomplete immunization** | Diphtheria |
| **Immunodeficiency** | Fungus |
| **Use of antibiotics** | *Candida* (thrush) |
| **What are some nonspecific symptoms of pharyngitis?** | Fever, sore throat, hoarseness of voice, rhinorrhea, cough, conjunctivitis, and cervical lymphadenopathy |

## CASE 16

*A 12-year-old girl presents to your clinic with complaints of sore throat for 3 days with associated cough and pea-sized bumps in her neck.*

| | |
|---|---|
| **On physical exam, if you found these findings, what agent would rise to the top of the list on your differential diagnosis?** | |
| **Pharyngeal erythema, tonsillar exudates, enlarged tonsils, lymphadenopathy, and hepatosplenomegaly** | Infectious mononucleosis viral pharyngitis |
| **Significant pharyngeal erythema and petechiae, white tonsillar exudates, tender anterior cervical lymphadenopathy, and scarlatiniform (sand paper-like) rash** | Streptococcal pharyngitis |
| **Pharyngeal or oral nodules or ulcers, conjunctivitis, and skin rash** | Enteroviral pharyngitis |

**You've completed your exam and are confident of the diagnosis below. What test will you order to confirm or strengthen your diagnosis?**

| | |
|---|---|
| *S. pyogenes* **pharyngitis** | Throat culture (diagnostic) and rapid streptococcal antigen detection tests |
| **Infectious mononucleosis** | Peripheral smear looking for more than 10% atypical lymphocytes, Monospot (heterophil antibodies), and EBV IgM antibody serology (best test) |

**You've made your diagnosis below. What's your treatment?**

| | |
|---|---|
| **Viral pharyngitis** | Symptomatic: analgesics and antipyretics |
| **GABHS pharyngitis** | Oral or IM penicillin V (oral erythromycin if PCN allergic) |

## CASE 17

*A 4-year-old Japanese child presents with temperature of 103°F for the last 5 days. On exam you find an erythematous rash, conjunctivitis, cervical adenopathy, and swollen hands and feet.*

| | |
|---|---|
| **What's your differential diagnosis?** | Kawasaki disease, scarlet fever, toxic shock, leptospirosis, Epstein-Barr virus, juvenile rheumatoid arthritis, measles, Rocky Mountain spotted fever, drugs, and Stevens-Johnson syndrome |
| **Which disease is most likely?** | Kawasaki disease |
| **Why?** | Child is younger than 5 years of age, Japanese (most often affected), and meets 2 of the criteria for the diagnosis |
| **Elaborate on the following criteria to make the diagnosis** | |
| **Fever** | Unexplained for at least 5 days |

| | |
|---|---|
| **Physical exam** | 4 of the following 5 symptoms are present: conjunctivitis, mucus membrane changes (strawberry tongue, dry cracked lips), cervical lymphadenopathy, rash, and changes in hands or feet with swelling or desquamation (usually occurs later if at all) |
| **What labs should you order and what do you expect to find on** | |
| **CBC?** | Leukocytosis with left shift, anemia, thrombocytosis |
| **CRP and ESR?** | Elevated |
| **LFTs?** | Elevated |
| **What additional tests do you need to order?** | CXR, EKG, echocardiogram |
| **Why?** | Kawasaki disease is a febrile illness associated with vasculitis of the coronary arteries (1/4 of cases) causing them to acutely thrombose or chronically stenose, putting the child at risk of a myocardial infarction. |
| **What is the treatment?** | Intravenous γ-globulin and salicylates |

## CASE 18

*A 4-year-old child comes to the ER with sudden onset of fever, sore throat, drooling, leaning forward with hand on knees with inspiratory stridor, and respiratory distress.*

| | |
|---|---|
| **What's your differential diagnosis?** | Epiglottitis, croup, pertussis, retropharyngeal abscess, foreign body, angioneurotic edema |
| **What diagnosis is most likely?** | Epiglottitis |

| | |
|---|---|
| **How is this presentation distinguished from that of croup?** | Children with croup usually have an associated upper respiratory infection; children with epiglottitis do not. |
| **What do you need to do first with this child?** | Get equipment ready for intubation or tracheostomy if needed. |
| **Should you examine the airway by using a tongue blade?** | No |
| **Why?** | Any examination or irritation of the airway may induce laryngospasm and complete airway obstruction. |
| **Is there a safe way to examine the airway?** | Yes |
| **How?** | Transport the patient sitting up to the OR for direct visualization of the epiglottis with a fiberoptic laryngoscope with intubation gear ready. |
| **What do you expect to see?** | Swollen cherry red epiglottis |
| **What radiographic image would support your diagnosis?** | Lateral neck x-ray showing the "thumbprint sign" of a swollen epiglottis |
| **Should the x-ray be ordered when the patient has respiratory distress?** | No, it delays setting up for and securing a stable airway. |
| **What infectious agents cause epiglottitis?** | *H. influenzae* type B (vaccine use has greatly decreased the incidence), *Streptococcus*, and *Staphylococcus* species |
| **How does it begin?** | As cellulites between the tongue base and epiglottis that displaces the epiglottis posteriorly |
| **The diagnosis has been made. What's the treatment?** | Intubation and IV cefuroxime |

## NEPHROLOGY

CASE 19

*A 6-year-old boy had a viral syndrome 1 week ago, was given aspirin, and now presents with fever, intractable vomiting, lethargy, and confusion.*

**What's your differential diagnosis?**

Encephalitis, meningitis, inherited metabolic disorders, drug intoxication, uncontrolled diabetes, Reye syndrome

**Pertinent positive physical exam findings include fever of 103°F, mild liver enlargement, no jaundice, fever, or focal neurological findings. Which diagnosis is most likely?**

Reye syndrome based on preceding viral illness, aspirin ingestion, then fever, vomiting, and altered mental status with above exam findings

**What illnesses is this associated with?**

Influenza A and B, and varicella (chicken pox). Other viruses have been implicated as well.

**What causes it?**

An acute syndrome of unknown etiology causing encephalopathy and fatty degeneration of the liver

**What causes the neurologic changes?**

Cerebral edema leading to increased intracranial pressure

**What labs should you order when suspecting Reye syndrome?**

CBC, Chem 8, LFTs, ammonia, coags (Pt, PTT, INR)

**What change do you expect to see in the following laboratory tests?**

**ALT and AST**

Markedly increased

**Total bilirubin and alkaline phosphatase**

Normal or slightly increased

**Ammonia**

Elevated

| | |
|---|---|
| **PT** | Prolonged |
| **Creatinine kinase and lactic dehydrogenase** | Increased |
| **Serum glucose** | May be low |
| **What prognostic significance does elevated ammonia and PT have?** | Increased risk of coma and coagulopathy, respectfully |
| **What diagnostic procedures might you consider?** | CSF studies, liver biopsy |
| **What CSF and liver biopsy findings are consistent with Reye syndrome?** | |
| **CSF** | Increased CSF pressure without leukocytosis (not an infectious process) |
| **Liver biopsy** | Foamy cytoplasm with microvesicular fat and severe mitochondrial injury |
| **How is Reye syndrome diagnosed?** | By history, physical exam, and lab findings. There is no specific test to make the diagnosis. |
| **How is Reye syndrome treated?** | Therapy is symptomatic and supportive. |

## MISCELLANEOUS DISORDERS

### CASE 20

*A 43-year-old woman delivers a baby with Down syndrome and your attending asks you to examine the infant and report what physical exam findings are consistent with the diagnosis.*

| | |
|---|---|
| **What will you be looking for on the** | |
| **Eyes?** | Speckled iris |
| **Nose?** | Broad bridged |

| | |
|---|---|
| **Face?** | Flattened, upward slanted palpebral fissures, epicanthal folds |
| **Mouth?** | High arched palate, protruding tongue |
| **Neck?** | Webbed |
| **4 hours after birth, the baby begins to vomit bile-stained emesis. What disorder do you suspect?** | Duodenal atresia because infants with Down syndrome are at a greater risk of this disorder |
| **What test will you order to confirm your diagnosis** | Abdominal x-ray |
| **What do you expect the report to read?** | Double bubble sign |
| **What is the treatment?** | Surgery |
| **The mother is distressed because no one ever told her she was going to have a child with Down syndrome and she does not want to have any more children with this kind of surprise. You inform her there are tests to screen and diagnose the syndrome prior to birth. Name the tests and values.** | |
| **Screening: Mother** | Abnormal triple screening test |
| | Decreased α-fetoprotein |
| | Decreased unconjugated estriol |
| | Increased human chorionic gonadotropin |
| **Diagnostic: Fetus** | Chromosomal analysis showing trisomy 21 |
| **Name the 3 ways in which trisomy occurs.** | An individual receiving 3 copies of a chromosome, a translocation, or a mosaicism |

| | |
|---|---|
| **The father pulls you aside and asks what other diseases may the child develop as a result of being diagnosed with Down syndrome. Name them by organ system:** | |
| **GI** | Duodenal atresia |
| | Hirshsprung disease |
| **Cardiac** | Atrioventricular canal |
| | Ventricular septal defect |
| | Patent ductus arteriosus |
| | Atrial septal defect |
| | Tetrology of Fallot |
| **Neurologic/cognitive** | Hypotonia and varying degrees of mental retardation |
| **Endocrine** | Hypothyroid (requires yearly TSH screening) |
| **The father asked what put their child at risk of this condition. What is your reply?** | Advanced maternal age is the major risk factor for having a child with Down syndrome (1/2000 age 20 and 1/20 age 45). |
| **What therapy will you recommend to ensure the child reaches his full potential?** | Therapy should be problem directed. Children with Down syndrome should receive the therapy and intervention to ensure that they reach their full potential. |

## CASE 21

*A 14-year-old girl presents complaining that all her girlfriends' periods began last year and she is worried that there is something wrong.*

| | |
|---|---|
| **What's your differential diagnosis?** | Imperforate hymen, mullerian agenesis, constitutional delay, Turner syndrome |

| | |
|---|---|
| **On a limited physical exam you find short stature, sparse pubic-axillary hair, and failure of development of secondary sex characteristics. What is your lead diagnosis in the differential now?** | Turner syndrome (TS) |
| **What would you expect to find on a complete physical exam?** | Webbing of neck, cubitus valgus, low hair line, low-set ears, micrognathia, shield chest with widespread nipples, short 4th metacarpals, lymphedema of feet or hands |
| **What lab tests should be ordered to support your diagnosis?** | Follicle-stimulating hormone (FSH) and Luteinizing hormone (LH) |
| **What impact does the disease have on these levels?** | Increased |
| **What does this signify?** | Ovarian failure |
| **What test do you order to confirm the diagnosis?** | A karyotype analysis |
| **What result do you expect?** | Absence or abnormality of an X chromosome, 45, XO |
| **What is the treatment for patients with TS?** | Sex steroid supplementation |
| **What additional imaging tests should you order now that the diagnosis has been made?** | Renal and cardiac ultrasound to detect anomalies |
| **Name the renal and cardiac disorders associated with TS.** | |
|     **Renal** | Horseshoe kidney, double collecting system |
|     **Cardiac** | Bicuspid aortic valve, aortic coarctation, aortic stenosis |

## MISCELLANEOUS CASES

A 6-month-old baby is crying excessively, has a bruise on her forehead, and has retinal hemorrhages evident on ophthalmologic exam. The mother is distraught and states she feels guilty because she dropped the child by accident when picking her up. What is the most likely diagnosis?

Shaken baby syndrome (a form of physical child abuse)

An 8-month-old child is brought in for her third visit in 2 weeks with poor weight gain, poor skin turgor, and no mittens or winter coat with a temperature of 40°F outside. What is the most likely diagnosis?

Neglect

A 6-year-old child has had repeated visits to the school administrators for truancy and poor scholastic performance. What is the most likely diagnosis?

Neglect

A 12-year-old girl returns to the clinic with recurrent abdominal pain, urinary tract infection, and trace amounts of vaginal bleeding. What is the most likely diagnosis?

Sexual abuse

When child abuse is suspected, what do you need to do first?

Contact child protective services with a full report (your legal obligation); do not allow child to return home.

**What additional workup is required for each type of abuse?**

    **Sexual**

Tests for gonorrhea, chlamydia, syphilis, and HIV even if genital exam is normal

    **Physical**

X-rays (complete skeletal survey)

**What is your basic treatment plan for all forms of child abuse?**

Contact social services, do not allow child to go home, treat any associated injuries or infections, and arrange counseling for child and family.

# Psychiatry

## PSYCHOSIS

CASE 1

*You're called to see a 17-year-old previously healthy female who returned from college after her dorm supervisor found her wandering in the hall talking to herself. When asked what was wrong, she said the dorm room numbers were code for others to inflict harm on her. Her roommates and dorm room neighbors deny any such intent.*

| | |
|---|---|
| **What should you be concerned about?** | Schizophrenia |
| **What's a brief differential diagnosis for schizophrenia?** | Bipolar disorder, schizoaffective disorder, and brief psychotic disorder |
| **What is the common age of onset for schizophrenia?** | Late teens to early 30s (she's 17) |
| **What causes it?** | Etiology unknown, but dopamine hyperactivity has been implicated (dopamine hypothesis) |
| **Describe the 5 subtypes of schizophrenia.** | |
|     **Paranoid** | Paranoid delusions, auditory hallucinations, and nonflat affect (best prognosis) |
|     **Catatonic** | Psychomotor disturbance ranging from excessive increase or decrease in activity, echolia, or mutism |
|     **Disorganized** | Disorganized speech and behavior, flat or inappropriate affect (worst prognosis) |

| | |
|---|---|
| **Undifferentiated** | Criteria not met for paranoid, catatonic, or disorganized |
| **Residual** | Period of persistent negative symptoms and/or mild positive symptoms after 1 acute episode of schizophrenia |
| **Which subtype is most likely in her?** | Paranoid schizophrenia |
| **How is the diagnosis made?** | Presence of symptoms, associated with social and occupational deterioration for at least 6 months |
| **What determines the type of treatment?** | Presence of positive or negative symptoms |
| **What are the positive symptoms?** | Delusions, hallucinations, disorganized speech or behavior, and catatonic behavior |
| **What are the negative symptoms?** | Flat affect apathy, anhedonia inattentiveness |
| **What is the first-line treatment for positive symptoms?** | Antipsychotic medications—haloperidol (higher potency for severely agitated or disruptive behavior) or chlorpromazine (lower potency) |
| **What is the mechanism of action for haloperidol and chlorpromazine?** | Dopamine receptor antagonists |
| **What is an alternative medication for patients with negative symptoms?** | Risperidone |
| **What medication is prescribed if patients fail first-line agents?** | Clozapine |
| **What is the dreaded complication of schizophrenia?** | Suicide |

## DISORDERS ORIGINATING IN CHILDHOOD

CASE 2

*A 5-year-old boy arrives at your family practice clinic after being reprimanded many times in the last 12 weeks for excessive talkativeness and inability to complete school classroom projects.*

| | |
|---|---|
| **What could the child have?** | Attention-deficit hyperactivity disorder (ADHD) |
| **What is ADHD?** | A disorder characterized by inattention, impulsiveness, and hyperactive behavior in young children often labeled as "troublemakers" |
| **What causes it?** | Etiology unknown, but depletion of the neurotransmitter dopamine has been implicated as well as prenatal substance abuse |
| **Which sex is it more common in?** | Male (4:1) |
| **Describe the following typical behaviors:** | |
| **Inattentive** | Inability to complete tasks (often in school); easily distracted or forgetful |
| **Impulsive** | Impatient and frequently interrupts |
| **Hyperactive** | Excessive talkativeness, restlessness, or fidgety behavior |
| **How is it diagnosed?** | Age <7 and symptoms present in 2 separate locations (e.g., school and home) |
| **So what's the next step with this child?** | Ask the mother about behavior in other settings. |
| **What is the first-line treatment for ADHD?** | Employ behavior management techniques |

| | |
|---|---|
| **What's the next step?** | Consider psychostimulants like methylphenidate (Ritalin) if necessary |
| **What are the side effects of Ritalin?** | Insomnia, depressed mood, irritability, tics, and decreased growth rate (higher doses) |

## ANXIETY

### CASE 3

*A patient's wife calls you concerned that her husband is worrying excessively about financial matters and local and world events and, as a result, has had little sleep for 9 months. She is not sure why he is so anxious.*

| | |
|---|---|
| **What could this patient have?** | Generalized anxiety disorder |
| **What are the main clinical features?** | Excessive, persistent, uncontrollable anxiety or apprehension about most daily events |
| **What additional symptoms may be present secondary to the anxiety?** | Difficulty concentrating, restlessness, easily fatigued, sleep disturbance, and muscle tension |
| **What lab tests are included in the workup to rule out anxiety secondary to a medical condition?** | Thyroid function tests, glucose, CBC, electrolytes, and calcium |
| **What basic cardiac study should be considered in the workup?** | EKG |
| **How is it diagnosed?** | Persistent anxiety that occurs most days for at least 6 months with at least 3 secondary symptoms |
| **What is the first-line therapy?** | Psychotherapy and relaxation techniques |
| **What is the second-line therapy?** | Anxiolytics (e.g., benzodiazepines and buspirone) |

## CASE 4

*A mother brings her 13-year-old child into the office complaining that he is obsessive about personal hygiene. She says it is not uncommon for her son to spend 20 minutes in the bathroom just washing his hands after using the bathroom. He is concerned about his repetitive hand washing, but has difficulty stopping.*

| | |
|---|---|
| **What is this presentation classic for?** | Obsessive compulsive disorder |
| **Define an obsession.** | Persistent intrusive thoughts, impulses, ideas, or images that cause significant anxiety and cannot be controlled |
| **Define a compulsion.** | A repeated mental or motor behavior performed to lessen anxiety, often follows obsession |
| **What are some examples of compulsions?** | Repetitive checking, washing, and counting |
| **How is it diagnosed?** | Recurrent obsessions and compulsions that cause significant distress. Patient must be aware that these do not make sense. |
| **What is the first-line medical therapy?** | Selective serotonin reuptake inhibitors (SSRIs) (e.g., fluvoxamine) |
| **What is the next medical therapy available?** | Tricyclic antidepressants (TCAs) (e.g., clomipramine) |
| **What additional therapy should be considered?** | Behavior modification techniques (e.g., systemic desensitization and flooding) |

## CASE 5

*A 25-year-old female presents after having repetitive episodes of intense fear with palpitations and sweating while driving on the expressway. It often happens while driving the speed limit during time periods other than rush hour. The intense fear of an accident causes her to pull over to the side of the road and rest for about 20 minutes. After 6 episodes, she is worried about additional attacks and the impact on her ability to function.*

**What disorder is most likely?**   Panic disorder

**How does it present?**   Often females 20 to 30 years old with recurrent, unexpected, discrete periods of intense fear or discomfort, with 4 or more panic symptoms and constant worry about having another attack

**Name some common panic attack symptoms.**   Palpitations, accelerated heart rate, sweating, shaking, shortness of breath, feeling of choking, chest discomfort, nausea, dizziness, fear of losing control or dying

**What associated cardiac disease might be found on physical exam?**   Mitral valve prolapse

**What laboratory test should you order and why?**   TSH to exclude thyroid disease

**How is it diagnosed?**   Recurrent attacks (at least 4 symptoms) with at least 1 month of associated anxiety

**What other disorder may occur with panic disorder?**   Agoraphobia

**Define agoraphobia.**   Intense fear of places or situations in which escape might be difficult or help may not be available if panic symptoms occur

**What medical treatments are used to treat panic attacks?**   TCAs (desipramine), monoamine oxidase inhibitors (phenelzine), SSRIs (fluoxetine), and benzodiazepines (alprazolam)

**What additional therapy should be considered?**   Cognitive-behavioral therapy (e.g., relaxation exercises and desensitization)

**What is the treatment for agoraphobia?**   Exposure therapy

CASE 6

A 55-year-old Vietnam veteran comes to your office complaining of difficulty sleeping owing to recurrent flashbacks to his bloody combat days after attending a veteran reunion. He awakes in a sweat with his heart pounding and has difficulty falling back to sleep.

| | |
|---|---|
| **What is this presentation consistent with?** | Post-traumatic stress disorder |
| **What is the main risk factor?** | Traumatic events (e.g., rape, assault, combat, and natural catastrophes) |
| **How does it present?** | Re-experience (recurrent hallucinations, illusions, or flashbacks of the event), increased arousal (anxiety, sleep disturbance, and hypervigilance), and avoidance of stimuli associated with the trauma |
| **How is it diagnosed?** | Presenting symptoms (above) lasting more than 1 month during which time patient must have experienced severe fear, hopelessness, or horror |
| **So, what is the key question for this patient?** | Duration of symptoms |
| **What is the treatment?** | Psychotherapy and TCAs (e.g., imiprimine) and SSRIs (e.g., fluoxetine) |
| **What is an alternative drug for imipramine?** | Phenelzine (monoamine oxidase inhibitor) |

CASE 7

A 29-year-old female comes to your office after experiencing excessive amounts of fear during public speaking events and now has considerable apprehension about future talks. Upon further questioning, you find out that she has also been fearful of large social functions like weddings since she was a teenager.

| | |
|---|---|
| **What is this most likely?** | Social phobia |
| **How does it present?** | Excessive, persistent fear of social or performance situations |
| **How is it diagnosed?** | History |
| **What is the first-line treatment?** | Behavioral therapy (desensitization, rehearsal) |
| **What is the second-line therapy?** | Selective serotonin reuptake inhibitors (SSRIs) (e.g., fluoxetine) or monoamine oxidase inhibitor (MAOI) (e.g., phenelzine) |
| **What medication may be useful if taken 30 minutes before performance situations?** | Propranolol |

## MOOD DISORDERS

### CASE 8

*You've met your girlfriend's mother multiple times and have noticed a signifi-cant variation in her behavior. Some days she sleeps in late, has decreased interest in her usual activities, and complains of fatigue. Other times she has high self-esteem, loves to travel, and works feverishly on her hobbies and goals. Everyone in your girlfriend's family says that's just the way she is.*

| | |
|---|---|
| **What is most likely wrong with her?** | Bipolar disorder |
| **What disorders comprise it?** | Mania (or hypomania) and major depression |
| **Describe features of a manic episode.** | Elevated self-esteem, decreased sleep, pressured speech, racing speech, flight of ideas, easily distracted, increased goal-directed activity, excess involvement in pleasurable activities like sex, spending, and travel |
| **How is a manic episode diagnosed?** | 3 to 4 of the above features lasting 1 week or severe enough to require hospitalization |

| | |
|---|---|
| **Define bipolar I disorder.** | At least 1 episode of mania with or without a major depressive episode (for description see respective section) |
| **Define bipolar II disorder.** | One or more hypomanic episodes plus one or more major depressive episodes (no history of manic episode) |
| **What medications may be used for rapid treatment of manic episodes?** | Benzodiazepines or antipsychotics |
| **What is the long-term treatment strategy?** | Psychotherapy, cognitive therapy, lithium (monitor levels closely due to toxic potential) |
| **What is a frequently tested side effect of lithium?** | Hypothyroidism |
| **What second-line drugs are available to treat mania?** | Carbamzepine and valproic acid |

## CASE 9

*A 44-year-old patient comes to your clinic for routine follow-up and you find out that he recently lost his job 6 months ago and is having a hard time finding work. He later remarks that he has been having difficulty sleeping, has decreased energy, and is not playing nearly as much golf as usual for the last 4–5 months.*

| | |
|---|---|
| **What diagnosis is most likely here?** | Adjustment disorder with depressed mood (ADDM) |
| **Why is it not major depression?** | ADDM presents with depressed or anxious mood within 3 months of identifiable stressor, lasting less than 6 months; mood change is excessive and/or impairs social/occupational functioning. |
| **What stressor did he have?** | Lost his job |
| **Name other common stressors preceding ADDM.** | Marital problems, divorce, moving, financial hardship, and criminal victim |

| | |
|---|---|
| **How is it diagnosed?** | History and presentation (as above) |
| **What is first-line therapy?** | Psychotherapy |
| **What is the treatment for severe anxiety?** | Short-term use of benzodiazepines |
| **What is the treatment for depressed mood?** | Antidepressants (use is controversial) |

## CASE 10

*A 44-year-old female presents with impaired sleep, decreased interest in typical activities, fatigue, and anorexia 3 months after her husband died in an auto accident. Her symptoms have not changed significantly over the last 3 months.*

| | |
|---|---|
| **What's in your differential diagnosis?** | Normal or complicated bereavement |
| **How do they both present?** | Sudden or delayed onset (up to a year) of depressive symptoms following loss of loved one after a traumatic event |
| **What are typical traumatic events?** | Sudden or traumatic death, death of a child, concurrent stress, insecure personality |
| **When does normal bereavement become complicated?** | When symptoms persist for >2 months |
| **What is the therapy?** | Bereavement therapy |
| **When should hospitalization be considered?** | If patient is at risk of suicide |
| **What are patients at risk for?** | Major depression and suicide |

## CASE II

*A 39-year-old male patient arrives at your office for his first visit after moving from another state. He has no specific complaints other than feeling depressed. This is no different than he has felt for years and he just goes on with his life. His last doctor referred him to a psychiatrist and diagnosed him with a milder form of depression, not major depression.*

| | |
|---|---|
| **What diagnosis most likely was it?** | Dysthymic disorder |
| **What is it?** | A chronic form of mild depression |
| **How does it present?** | Almost continuous depressed mood and symptoms most of the time for at least 2 years |
| **Name some common depressive symptoms.** | Change in appetite, sleep disturbances, fatigue, low self-esteem, decreased concentration, and feelings of hopelessness |
| **How is it diagnosed?** | History and presentation |
| **What is the treatment?** | Psychotherapy and antidepressants |

## CASE 12

*A 30-year-old previously healthy female comes to your office with her husband complaining that she has no energy, no interest in playing her beloved piano, feelings of worthlessness, sleeping all the time, difficulty concentrating, and had 10-pound weight loss. The remainder of her review of systems and physical exam is normal.*

| | |
|---|---|
| **What's the differential diagnosis?** | Major depressive episode, bipolar disorder, dysthymic disorder, depression secondary to undiagnosed medical condition |
| **Which is most likely?** | Major depressive disorder |
| **In what age range does major depression typically appear?** | 20–50 (she's 30) |
| **What pneumonic can be used to remember the criteria to diagnose major depression?** | SIGMECAPS |
| **Describe what each letter represents.** | |
| **Sleep** | Insomnia or hypersomnia |

| | |
|---|---|
| **Interest** | Marked decrease in interest and pleasure in most activities |
| **Guilt** | Feeling worthless or inappropriate guilt |
| **Mood** | Depressed mood most of the day, nearly every day |
| **Energy** | Fatigue or low energy nearly every day |
| **Concentration** | Decreased concentration or increased indecisiveness |
| **Appetite** | Increased or decreased or weight gain or weight loss |
| **Psychomotor** | Psychomotor agitation or retardation |
| **Suicidality** | Recurrent thoughts of death, suicidal ideation, suicide plan, suicide attempt |
| **How is it diagnosed?** | 5 or more of the above criteria for at least 2 weeks; 1 symptom must be depressed mood or loss of interest or pleasure and no history of manic episodes. |
| **What lab tests should be ordered to rule out major depression secondary to another medical condition?** | CBC, electrolytes, liver function test, urinalysis, thyroid function tests, and drug screen |
| **What radiographic studies may be ordered to exclude intracranial causes?** | CT or MRI |
| **What is the treatment for milder cases?** | Psychotherapy (e.g., supportive, cognitive-behavioral, and brief interpersonal therapies) |
| **What additional treatment is available?** | Pharmacotherapy [e.g., SSRIs, TCAs, and monoamine oxidase inhibitors (MAOIs)] |
| **What 2 neurotransmitters have been implicated in major depression?** | Norepinephrine and serotonin |

| | |
|---|---|
| **What determines which medication is prescribed?** | Medication history and side-effect profile of the medication |
| **What is considered an adequate trial of a medicine?** | 4 weeks at maximum recommended dose |
| **In which patients are SSRIs (e.g., fluoxetine, sertraline, and paroxetine) especially useful?** | Cardiac disease patients (minimal risk of cardiac complications) and patients at risk of suicide (overdose less likely to be fatal) |
| **What are the common side effects of SSRIs?** | GI side effects, sexual dysfunction, and appetite suppression |
| **Name some commonly prescribed TCAs.** | Amitriptyline, nortriptyline, imipramine, desipramine, and doxepin |
| **What are the side effects of TCAs?** | Anticholinergic side effects (e.g., dry mouth, constipation, cardiac arrhythmias), sexual dysfunction, and potential for fatal overdose |
| **Name 3 MAOIs.** | Phenelzine, tranylcypromine, and isocarboxazid |
| **When are MAOIs useful?** | In patients with excessive anxiety (including panic symptoms) or with mild atypical depression (e.g., increased sleep, increased appetite) |
| **What is the main side effect of MAOIs?** | Hypotension |
| **What are patients taking MAOIs at risk for if they eat foods containing tyramine?** | Tyramine hypertensive crisis which could lead to death |
| **What foods contain tyramine?** | Aged cheese, red wine, and aged/processed meats |
| **When should electroconvulsive therapy be considered?** | Patients who fail pharmacotherapy or who are acutely suicidal |

| | |
|---|---|
| **When should a patient be hospitalized?** | When it has been determined that the patient has a significant risk of harming himself or others (e.g., those with command auditory hallucinations) because of their mental disorder |

## CASE 13

*A 32-year-old 1-week postpartum female who recently resigned from work to stay home with her newly born son develops depressive symptoms.*

| | |
|---|---|
| **What's the differential diagnosis for postpartum mood disorders?** | Postpartum blues, postpartum depression, puerperal psychosis |
| **What risk factor for postpartum depression does she have?** | Unemployment |
| **Name other major risk factors for postpartum depression.** | Previous mood disorder, particularly postpartum; social stresses (e.g., marital conflict, limited social support); infant health problems or irritability |
| **What causes them?** | A combination of genetic predisposition and physiologic changes (e.g., decreased estrogen, progesterone, and cortisol) and psychosocial factors |
| **How do they present?** | |
| **Postpartum blues** | Mild depressive symptoms that develop in the first week postpartum and resolve in the second week; very common—up to 85% of postpartum women) |
| **Postpartum depression** | A major depressive episode occurring within 4 weeks of childbirth; common—up to 15% of postpartum women |
| **Puerperal psychosis** | A psychotic disorder developing in the weeks postpartum; usually presents as a mood episode with psychotic symptoms; rare—1/1000–1/1500 postpartum women; medical emergency |

| | |
|---|---|
| **Which two are more likely in her?** | Postpartum depression or blues (mild depressive symptoms) |
| **What's your next step?** | Apply SIGMECAPS pneumonic for major depression and if 5 or more present diagnosis is made, otherwise postpartum blues is diagnosed |
| **What is the treatment for postpartum depression?** | Psychotherapy (interpersonal or cognitive behavioral) and medication; ECT for severe symptoms |
| **What medications are used to treat postpartum depression?** | SSRIs are first-line, TCAs are a frequent second choice |
| **What specific concerns are there with postpartum drug therapy?** | All psychoactive medications are secreted into breast milk; effect on infant is generally unclear. Breast-feeding is contraindicated with lithium. |
| **How is the mother at risk?** | Poor parenting skills, plus the usual risks of depression (e.g., relationship and work problems, suicide) |
| **How is the infant at risk?** | Increased risk of retarded cognitive, behavioral, and emotional development, child abuse and neglect, and infanticide |

## SOMATOFORM DISORDERS

CASE 14

*A 27-year-old healthy female comes to your office for her yearly exam. During the examination you find out she plans to have a second rhinoplasty on her nose. No physical or cosmetic defects are apparent on the exam. She is adamant that the slope and angle of her left nostril is abnormal and is of significant concern thus warranting repeat surgery.*

| | |
|---|---|
| **What do you think?** | She may have body dysmorphic disorder (BDD). |

| | |
|---|---|
| **Describe it.** | Gradual onset of excessive preoccupation with an imagined defect in appearance that causes significant distress and psychosocial impairment |
| **How will you diagnose it?** | History and presentation |
| **What is the treatment strategy?** | Noninvasive treatment of any medical disorder along with psychotherapy and medication trial |
| **What medications may be useful?** | Fluoxetine (first-line drug) and clomipramine (second-line drug); if refractory, try pimozide (an antipsychotic) |
| **What are patients at risk of?** | Major depression; up to 60% of BDD patients have major depressive disorder |
| **When is hospitalization required?** | Severe depression with suicide risk (up to 1/3 of BDD patients attempt suicide) |

## CASE 15

*At the beginning of your general neurology service month you are signed out a patient by one of your peers after an extensive workup. The patient, a 33-year-old female, has been worked up for complaints of bilateral lower extremity weakness, paresthesias, and right ear deafness that developed after hearing her brother was killed in a motor vehicle accident. Extensive neurologic workup has been negative. Neurologist states that the symptoms do not correlate with any known organic disease patterns. The patient is indifferent to the news and says "I guess I'll just have to go home and live with it."*

| | |
|---|---|
| **Before being discharged, what else should be done?** | Psychiatry consult |
| **Why?** | High suspicion for conversion disorder |
| **How does it present?** | Loss or alteration in physical functioning, usually neurologic (e.g., paralysis, aphonia, seizure, blindness, deafness); an acute stressor precedes the symptoms |

| | |
|---|---|
| **Why does it occur?** | Redirection of an unconscious psychological conflict or stressor into physical symptoms |
| **How is it diagnosed?** | By the presence of symptoms causing significant impairment without medical explanation and with inciting psychological stress |
| **What is the treatment?** | Psychotherapy and reassurance |
| **What's the recurrence rate of symptoms?** | 25% will have another episode |

## CASE 16

*A 33-year-old female with history of multiple atypical subcutaneous infections returns to the hospital again for complaints of multiple circular points of erythema around a pinpoint puncture site. She is afebrile and vital signs are normal. The cultures are back from her prior hospitalization for the same problem and they reveal a polymicrobial flora consistent with stool. Later, her husband arrives with a dirty syringe that he found under their bed.*

| | |
|---|---|
| **What's your differential diagnosis?** | Factitious disorder (a.k.a. Munchausen syndrome) and malingering |
| **How do they present?** | Intentionally produced or feigned signs and symptoms of a medical or psychiatric illness often resulting in multiple hospitalizations |
| **What distinguishes malingering from factitious disorder?** | In malingering, patient assumes sickness for external reward (most often money) |
| **How are they diagnosed?** | History, presentation, and evidence of feigned or self-induced illness |
| **What is the treatment?** | No effective therapy known; avoid unnecessary procedures and hospitalizations |

## CASE 17

*A 25-year-old graduate student presents to your office to follow up the results of the CT head taken last week for atypical headache. For the last 7 months, she was sure she had brain cancer and took several days off work even though her headaches were mild and had no neurologic examination findings to suspect underlying malignancy. When told of the results, she questions the validity of the study because she states she is sure she has a brain tumor. When asked about her headache, she says it comes and goes.*

| | |
|---|---|
| **What disorder might she have?** | Hypochondriasis |
| **How does it present?** | Preoccupation with fear of getting or having a serious disease; the preoccupation causes significant distress or impairs functioning |
| **How is it diagnosed?** | Persistence of the preoccupation >6 months despite medical evaluation and reassurance |
| **What is the treatment?** | Regularly scheduled office visits followed by psychotherapy |

## CASE 18

*A 33-year-old female presents to your office after being evaluated by 3 other primary care physicians and multiple specialists. She has consistently complained about recurring multiple points of pain on her body, nausea, abdominal pain, menstrual irregularities, and anxiety for over 6 years. Prior medical records indicate an extensive and complete workup with no identifiable medical illness.*

| | |
|---|---|
| **What's your differential diagnosis?** | Somatization disorder, somatoform disorder, conversion disorder, pain disorder, factitious disorder |
| **Which is most likely?** | Somatization disorder |

| | |
|---|---|
| **Why?** | Multiple medical complaints requiring treatment or impairing functioning, starting before 30 years old, and persisting over several years is consistent with the diagnosis. |
| **Name some common medical complaints.** | Pain, GI disturbance, menstrual irregularities, sexual symptoms, and pseudoneurologic symptoms |
| **What's the workup?** | Symptom-specific diagnostic workup if not already done in past |
| **How is it diagnosed?** | A history of pain in 4 sites plus other symptoms in 3 areas: GI (2 symptoms), sexual, and neurological without medical explanation for the symptoms; some symptoms develop before age 30 |
| **What is the treatment?** | Regular office visits; no laboratory evaluation or procedures without clear indications; psychiatry if patient amenable (usually not) |

## EATING DISORDERS

### CASE 19

*A 15-year-old female presents for her yearly physical exam required to play high school sports. Since last year, she has lost 18 pounds, appears ill, and complains of fatigue. Physical exam reveals a cachectic appearance with parotid gland swelling, dental erosions, and calluses on the dorsal aspect of her right hand. Her heart, lung, and abdomen exam is normal except for a scaphoid abdomen.*

| | |
|---|---|
| **What's your differential diagnosis?** | Anorexia nervosa (AN) or bulimia nervosa (BN) |
| **By history, which is more likely?** | Anorexia nervosa |
| **Why?** | Profound weight loss and cachectic appearance suggest AN. |

| | |
|---|---|
| **Name another way AN may present.** | Amenorrhea |
| **Name the two types of AN.** | Restricting type and binge-eating/purging type |
| **What clues on physical exam suggest the binge-eating/ purging type?** | Parotid gland swelling, hand calluses, and dental erosions |
| **What physical symptoms may be present in patients with AN?** | Constipation, abdominal pain, cold intolerance, lethargy, or excess energy |
| **What physical signs are often present in patients with AN?** | Severe cachexia, hypotension, hypothermia, xerosis, lanugo, bradycardia, parotid gland swelling, edema, dental enamel erosion, calluses on dorsum of hand |
| **What labs should be included in the workup?** | Comprehensive metabolic panel, serum albumin, and CBC |
| **What laboratory abnormalities may be seen in patients with AN?** | Anemia, leukopenia, hypokalemia, hypochloremic metabolic alkalosis, and hypoalbuminemia |
| **What additional test should be considered?** | EKG |
| **What are the psychological criteria necessary to diagnose AN?** | An extreme fear of gaining weight or of getting fat, and a distortion of perception of one's weight |
| **What medical complications are patients with AN at risk for?** | Cardiac arrhythmias, prolonged QT intervals, decreased left ventricular mass, gastric/intestinal dilatation, osteoporosis, sick euthyroid syndrome, cognitive dysfunction |
| **How is AN managed?** | Management of medical complications if present, including hospitalization for severe cases; family and behavioral psychotherapy; medicine may be helpful, e.g., chlorpromazine, cyproheptadine, and fluoxetine |

## CASE 21

A 15-year-old previously healthy female presents to your office after encouragement from her dentist after finding atypical erosions of her teeth enamel that cannot be explained by any dental disease. She's adamant that her dental hygiene is not a problem. The patient is very concerned about this because she prides herself on her appearance, figure, and weight. She wants to know what is causing it and how to reverse it.

| | |
|---|---|
| **What's your differential diagnosis?** | AN, BN |
| **What prior physical exam value is most useful is distinguishing these before taking additional history?** | Body weight |
| **What body weight trend is characteristic of BN?** | Weight maintained, or slight gain (AN typically has weight loss) |
| **Her weight has increased 2 pounds over the past 6 months; which diagnosis do you suspect?** | BN |
| **What is the classic presentation for BN?** | Recurrent binge eating followed by self-induced vomiting to prevent weight gain |
| **What's the name given to this type of BN?** | Purging type |
| **What are some other inappropriate nonpurging-type behaviors used to prevent weight gain in BN?** | Laxative abuse, fasting, excessive exercise |
| **What physical signs are associated with BN?** | Normal weight; with vomiting: erosion of dental enamel, scars/calluses on hand used to induce vomiting, parotid gland enlargement |
| **What lab values may be used to support the diagnosis?** | Chem 8 and amylase |

| | |
|---|---|
| **What lab abnormalities may be found with BN?** | Electrolyte disturbances, metabolic alkalosis and elevated serum amylase with vomiting, metabolic acidosis with laxative abuse |
| **What psychological symptom is necessary to diagnose BN?** | One's self-esteem is excessively influenced by one's body shape or weight (she admitted to this on presentation) |
| **What is the first-line therapy used in BN?** | Psychotherapy, particularly cognitive-behavioral |
| **What type of medication may be useful?** | Antidepressants |

## COGNITIVE DISORDERS

### CASE 22

*A 72-year-old male with history of HTN, CAD, and BPH with recurrent urinary tract infections (UTIs) is brought to the ER on Sunday by his daughter for sudden onset of confusion within the last 24 hours. Prior to being unaware of his surroundings and thinking it was 1965, he was performing his usual activities. He only complained to his daughter that he thought his prostate was acting up again and he wanted to go the doctor on Monday morning. He asked his daughter a day earlier for some Tylenol to help ease his pain with urination.*

| | |
|---|---|
| **Is this delirium or dementia?** | Delirium |
| **Describe the typical presentation of** | |
|     **Delirium** | Abrupt onset with fluctuating course with impaired consciousness and decreased attention |
|     **Dementia** | Insidious onset of impaired short-term memory; alert |
| **What are common causes of delirium?** | DELERIUMS: **D**rugs, **E**ndocrine, **L**ow $O_2$ (cardiac/stroke), **E**lectrolytes, **R**etention of stool or urine, **I**nfection, **U**ndernutrition/malnourished, **M**etabolic, **S**ubdural hematoma (head injury) |

| | |
|---|---|
| **What is most likely causing his delirium?** | UTI secondary to urinary stasis secondary to BPH |
| **What other factor should be addressed based on his history?** | MI (history of CAD) |
| **What tests would be most useful in this patient?** | UA, cardiac enzymes (CK-MB, troponin), EKG |
| **What tests are useful when the diagnosis is unclear?** | |
|     **Drugs** | Toxicology screen |
|     **Endocrine** | TSH |
|     **Low O$_2$** | Pulse ox, cardiac workup (EKG, cardiac enzymes), CBC (anemia) |
|     **Electrolytes** | Chem 8, magnesium, phosphorus |
|     **Retention** | KUB (assess stool), bladder scan or straight catherization (urinary retention) |
|     **Infection** | WBC |
|     **Undernutrition** | Albumin, prealbumin |
|     **Subdural hematoma (SDH)** | CT head |
| **What are the nursing approaches to a delirious patient?** | A quiet environment with decreased stimulation, frequent orientation, and reassurance by family and staff, close observation for agitation or impaired judgment, and minimal use of physical restraints |
| **What are the medical approaches to management?** | Identification and correction of contributing factors, nutritional support, sedation with high-potency antipsychotics |

## CASE 23

*A 68-year-old alert male with history of hyperlipidemia and type 2 diabetes mellitus presents with his wife with no complaints. His wife, however, says her husband frequently forgets what she has told him, often misplaces things, is easily agitated, gets lost away from home, and has difficulty balancing the checkbook. This has slowly been getting worse over the last year.*

| | |
|---|---|
| **What's the most likely diagnosis?** | Dementia |
| **How does it present?** | Progressive loss of previously acquired cognitive skills and judgment |
| **What's in the differential diagnosis for dementia?** | (1) Alzheimer disease (AD) |
| | (2) Brain cancer |
| | (3) Infection [AIDS, neurosyphilis, progressive multifocal leukoencephalopathy (PML)] |
| | (4) Metabolic (EtOH, hypothyroidism, $B_{12}$ and thiamine deficiency) |
| | (5) Organ failure (dialysis dementia, Wilson disease) |
| | (6) Vascular disorder [chronic subdural hematoma (SDH)] |
| | (7) Normal pressure hydrocephalus |
| | (8) Adverse drug effects |
| | (9) Depression (pseudodementia) |
| **What noncognitive symptom does this patient have that suggests AD?** | Agitation |
| **What other noncognitive symptoms may AD patients present with?** | Depression, anxiety, hallucinations, delusions, and sleep disturbances |

| | |
|---|---|
| **What additional history and physical exam information should be obtained at a minimum?** | Review medications he's taking that may cause mental status changes, depression screen, and on physical examination look for signs of metabolic disturbance or focal neurologic deficits |
| **What basic labs should be ordered in the workup to exclude secondary causes of dementia?** | CBC, Chem 8, glucose, liver and thyroid function tests, serum vitamin $B_{12}$ |
| **What if syphilis is suspected?** | Venereal Disease Research Laboratory (VDRL) and Rapid plasma realign (RPR) |
| **When would a lumbar puncture be warranted?** | Signs of cancer (weight loss, focal neurologic deficits), infection (fever, chills, nuchal rigidity), or rapid progression of symptoms |
| **What's the best test to rule out hydrocephalus, mass lesions, and SDH?** | CT scan or MRI of brain |
| **The above results are normal. What's your presumptive diagnosis?** | Alzheimer disease |
| **Is this surprising?** | No, it accounts for over 50% of new dementia cases. |
| **What are the risk factors for AD?** | Increasing age, family history, female gender, head injury, and lower education level |
| **Which chromosomes have been implicated in cases of familial AD?** | Chromosomes 1, 14, 19, and 21 |
| **What cognitive test should you order to confirm the diagnosis of dementia?** | Mini mental status examination (MMSE) |
| **What does the MMSE test?** | Orientation, attention, memory, and language |

| | |
|---|---|
| **How is the diagnosis of Alzheimer dementia made?** | By brain autopsy showing intracellular neurofibrillary tangles and neurotic (β-amyloid) plaques |
| **What nonpharmacological treatment modalities are useful in AD?** | Establishing a daily routine with familiar surroundings and support services for the caregiver, e.g., social services, education, counseling |
| **What drug treatment may improve cognitive symptoms in AD?** | Cholinesterase inhibitors, e.g., donepezil |

## PERSONALITY DISORDERS

### CASE 24

*A 45-year-old male comes to your office after an extensive medical and psychiatric workup for a long-standing abnormal pattern of behavior that has significantly impaired his ability to function normally in society. His workup to date is negative for any known medical disorder and the psychiatrist has just ruled out any specific psychiatric disease.*

| | |
|---|---|
| **What type of disorder does your patient have?** | Personality disorder (PD) |
| **Define a PD.** | A chronic pattern of behavior that is not due to another medical or psychiatric condition, e.g., a mood disorder that causes mental distress to the patient or impairs his social interactions and/or occupational functioning |
| **Describe the typical presentation for** | |
| **Paranoid PD** | Extensive and excessive suspiciousness and distrust of others |
| **Schizoid PD** | Socially isolated and emotionally cold |
| **Schizotypal PD** | Odd thinking, eccentric behavior, and social discomfort |

| | |
|---|---|
| **Antisocial PD** | Frequent disregard for social norms and for interests of others; often lacks remorse |
| **Borderline PD** | Unstable with mood swings, rocky relationships, and anger-control and impulse-control problems |
| **Histrionic PD** | Excessive attention-seeking and dramatic behavior |
| **Narcissistic PD** | Self-centered and insensitive to others |
| **Avoidant PD** | Inhibited with low self-esteem and excessive fear of rejection |
| **Dependent PD** | Passive and submissive with difficulty making decisions and fear of being left on one's own |
| **Obsessive-compulsive PD** | Perfectionist with a preoccupation with order and control |
| **What psychological tests may be helpful in assessing personality?** | The Minnesota multiphasic personality inventory (an objective personality test) and the Rorschach test and thematic apperception test (2 personality tests) |
| **Are PDs treated?** | Most are not treated because the patient is comfortable with the behaviors and they do not cause the patient significant distress. |
| **When should PDs be treated?** | When they cause a patient significant distress |
| **What treatments are available for PD?** | Psychotherapy and medication |
| **What medications may be used in the following situations?** | |
| **Psychosis and near-delusional thinking** | Antipsychotics |
| **Depression/anxiety** | Antidepressants |

# Appendix

**Table A-1. Immunizations**

| | Birth | 1 mo | 2 mos | 1-4 mos | 4 mos | 6 mos | 6-18 mos | 12-15 mos | 12-18 mos | 15-18 mos | 4-6 yrs | 11-12 yrs | 11-16 yrs | 6 mos to 18 yrs |
|---|---|---|---|---|---|---|---|---|---|---|---|---|---|---|
| HBV | X | X | | | | | X | | | | | | | |
| DTP | | | X | | X | X | | | | X | X | | | |
| HiB | | | X | | X | X | | | | | | | | |
| Polio (IPV) | | | X | | X | | | | X | | | | | |
| MMR | | | | | | | | X | | | X or | X | | |
| Td | | | | | | | | | | | | | X | |
| Varicella | | | | | | | | | X | | | | | |

337

## Table A–2. Growth and Development Chart

| | Sleep Position | Developmental Progress | Motor Skills | Social Skills | Communication Skills | Start Solids | Lead Testing | Temper Tantrums | Cognitive Skills | Language Skills | Toilet Training | Night Terrors |
|---|---|---|---|---|---|---|---|---|---|---|---|---|
| New-born | Supine | | | | | | | | | | | |
| 2–4 wks | | Raises head slightly, blinks in response to light, focuses and follows with eyes, and responds to sound by quickly turning toward noise | | | | | | | | | | |
| 2 mos | | Temporarily holds head erect, briefly holds rattle, tracks and follows objects, looks at faces and responds to sound, coos, and has a social smile | | | | | | | | | | |

| Age | | | |
|---|---|---|---|
| 4 mos | • Holds head erect<br>• No head lag when pulling to a sitting position<br>• Raises body using arms in prone position<br>• May roll one or both ways<br>• May support weight on legs<br>• Reaches for and grabs objects<br>• Puts hands together | Same as Communication Skills | • Tracks and follows objects visually to 180°<br>• Coos reciprocally<br>• Blows bubbles<br>• Makes "raspberry" sounds<br>• Smiles readily<br>• May laugh or squeal<br>• Differentiates individuals | 4–6 months solids are introduced; start with rice cereal. Foods to avoid till over 1 yr:<br>1. Honey<br>2. Corn syrup<br>3. Nuts<br>4. Strawberries<br>5. Chocolate<br>6. Egg whites<br>7. Cow's milk |
| 6 mos | • Holds head high when prone<br>• Holds head steady when pulled to a sit<br>• Rolls over both ways<br>• Sits with support<br>• Uses raking grasp to grab objects<br>• Transfers objects from one hand to the other | • Takes initiative in vocalizing or babbling at others<br>• Imitates sounds<br>• Smiles<br>• Laughs<br>• Coos to initiate social contact<br>• Recognizes parents<br>• Shows pleasure and excitement with interaction with parents | | |

(Continued)

**Table A-2. Growth and Development Chart (continued)**

| Sleep Position | Developmental Progress | Motor Skills | Social Skills | Communication Skills | Start Solids | Lead Testing | Temper Tantrums | Cognitive Skills | Language Skills | Toilet Training | Night Terrors |
|---|---|---|---|---|---|---|---|---|---|---|---|
| 9 mos | | • Sits well<br>• Crawls or creeps on hands<br>• May begin cruising furniture<br>• Begins to use pincer grasp<br>• Feeds self<br>• Bangs objects together | • Enjoys games: peek-a-boo and pat-a-cake<br>• May react to unfamiliar adults with fear or anxiety | • Responds to name<br>• Understands a few words: "no" and "bye-bye"<br>• Imitates vocalizations<br>• Babbles using several syllables | | | | | | | |
| 12 mos | | • Sits well<br>• Crawls<br>• Pulls self up and walks with support<br>• Feeds self<br>• Mature pincer grasp | • Plays games: peek-a-boo and pat-a-cake<br>• Waves bye-bye<br>• Looks at books<br>• Points at and names body parts or animals<br>• Follows simple commands<br>• Likes to play with adult-type objects such as phone or brush | • Uses mama and dada correctly<br>• Has 3–5 additional words | | Screening should begin at 1 year and be repeated again after 2 | | | | | |
| 15 mos | | • Feeds self with fingers or spoon<br>• Scribbles with crayons | • Shows functional understanding of objects (talks on toy | • Says 5–15 words<br>• Uses jargon<br>• Communicates | | | • Occur between 15 and 30 months | | | | |

| Age | Motor | Language | Social/Emotional |
|---|---|---|---|
| | • Stacks 2 blocks | with gestures<br>• Points to 1–2 body parts on request<br>• Understands simple commands<br>• Listens to stories<br>• Points to designated pictures in a book<br>• Communicates pleasure and displeasure | phone)<br>• Gives and takes toys<br>• Plays games with parents<br>• Tests parental rules or limits<br><br>• Normal ways for children to express frustration<br>• Occur as they strive to gain independence |
| 18 mos | • Walks quickly<br>• May run<br>• Walks up stairs with 1 hand held<br>• Walks backwards<br>• Eats with spoon and fork<br>• Stacks blocks<br>• Scribbles with crayons | • Understands commands<br>• Points to body parts<br>• May put 2 words together | • Knows location of objects that have been hidden<br>• Plays pretend games such as drinking from empty cup<br>• Hugs a doll<br>• Talks on the phone |

*(Continued)*

**Table A-2. Growth and Development Chart (*continued*)**

| Sleep Position | Developmental Progress | Motor Skills | Social Skills | Communication Skills | Start Solids | Lead Testing | Temper Tantrums | Cognitive Skills | Language Skills | Toilet Training | Night Terrors |
|---|---|---|---|---|---|---|---|---|---|---|---|
| 2 yrs | | • Running<br>• Jumping in place<br>• Walks up and down stairs<br>• Throws a ball overhead<br>• Opens doors<br>• Stacks blocks<br>• Imitates a vertical line<br>• Uses spoon and fork | • Imitates adults<br>• Parallel play with other kids<br>• Dresses and brushes teeth with help<br>• Feeds self | | | | | • Begins to create a means to accomplish a desired goal, i.e., pulls a chair to a cabinet and retrieves hidden object | • Greater than 50-word vocabulary<br>• Speaks several 2-word phrases<br>• Follows single and 2-step commands<br>• Listens to short stories<br>• Uses pronouns | | |
| 3 yrs | | • Jumps in place<br>• Kicks a ball<br>• Pedals tricycle<br>• Walks up stairs with alternating gait<br>• Scribbles<br>• Copies a circle<br>• Puts on some clothing | • Knows name, age, and sex<br>• Enjoys interactive play<br>• Participates in pretend play<br>• May be oppositional or destructive | • Speech is at least 75% intelligible<br>• Uses short sentences<br>• Asks questions such as "why" and "what's that"<br>• Understands prepositions and | | | | | | • Occurs between 18 and 30 months<br>• By age 3 about 90% are bowel-trained | |

| Age | | | | |
|---|---|---|---|---|
| | • Stacks 8 blocks | some adjectives | | and 85% are dry during daytime with 60–70% dry at night |
| 4 yrs | • Hops and balances on 1 foot<br>• Draws a circle and a cross<br>• Cuts with scissors<br>• Draws a person with 3–6 body parts | • Engages in interactive pretend play<br>• May have an imaginary friend<br>• May not differentiate reality from fantasy<br>• Brushes teeth<br>• Able to button and zip<br>• Toilet trained | • Extensive vocabulary<br>• Speech fully intelligible to strangers<br>• Uses full sentences with at least 6 words<br>• Asks questions such as "why" and "when"<br>• Recognizes some letters in the alphabet | • When counseling a parent:<br>• Child-size potty seat<br>• Modeling by parents and siblings<br>• Cooperation and success should be rewarded with praise<br>• Avoid punishment or shame in dealing with accidents<br>• Present in preschool and early school age<br>• Children cry inconsolably and appear terrified, confused, and glassy eyed |

# Index